# BECOME A VEGETARIAN
## *In Five Easy Steps!*

# BECOME A VEGETARIAN
## In Five Easy Steps!

by
Christine H. Beard

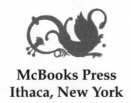

**McBooks Press**
**Ithaca, New York**

**A Word of Caution**
The information in this book should not be taken as professional advice for your personal medical situation. A substantial change in diet can alter your reaction to certain medications, so if you are ill or on medication, it is important that you not change your diet without supervision from your physician.

Library of Congress Cataloging-in-Publication Data

Beard, Christine H.
    Become a vegetarian in five easy steps! / by Christine H. Beard.
      p.    cm.
    Includes bibliographical references and index.
    ISBN 0-935526-25-0.
    1. Vegetarianism.    2. Diet.    I. Title.
  TX392.B35     1996
  641.5´636--dc20

Distributed to the book trade by:
Login Trade, 1436 West Randolph, Chicago, IL 60607, 312-432-7600.

Additional copies of this book may be ordered from any bookstore or directly from McBooks Press, 908 Steam Mill Road, Ithaca, NY 14850. Please include $3.00 postage and handling with mail orders. New York State residents must add 8% sales tax. All McBooks Press publications can also be ordered by calling toll-free 1-888-BOOKS11 (1-888-266-5711).

Printed in the United States of America

9 8 7 6 5 4 3 2 1

# Dedication

I dedicate this book to all those beings, both human and other-than-human, who showed me the way so that I might, in turn, show others.

"The means we choose dictate the ends we achieve."
Gloria Steinem
*Moving Beyond Words*

# Acknowledgments

Uncounted thanks to my editor, Wendy Skinner, who has given me invaluable encouragement and advice throughout the revisions for this book. I also wish to thank all those anonymous people who staffed the phone lines of the organizations I contacted for information. Their cheerful, generous assistance was much appreciated.

# Table of Contents

# Changing Habits, Changing Lives

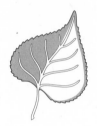

## *Overview*

A major change is under way in America. After decades of eating a diet based on animal products, people from all walks of life are waking up to the possibilities of a diet based on plants. By picking up this book, you are participating in a revolution. You are joining millions of other people in discovering the joys of a vegetarian diet.

*Become a Vegetarian in Five Easy Steps!* is designed to gently guide you in your transition from an animal-centered diet to a plant-based diet. This is not a book about why to become a vegetarian. There are already many excellent books available on that subject. Instead, it is a book about *how*.

The core of this book is a Five Step process designed to teach you how to change the foods you eat. Before going through the Five Steps, you will be asked to answer some questions to help you define your goals. Once you have completed the Five Steps, you will want to move on to the remaining chapters, which will help you fine-tune your new diet. The book concludes with a detailed list of vegetarian resources which you can use for many years to come.

How long it takes you to move through the entire Five Step process is up to you. You can complete the Five Steps over the course of several days (the "cold tofu" approach), or you can do one step and then wait a week or a month before going to the next (the "gradual" approach). You can also combine the two approaches. By proceeding through the steps in the manner suggested in the text, you can look forward to becoming a full-fledged vegetarian somewhere from one week to six months after you begin!

## *Embracing Change*

People are changing their diets for many different reasons—such as personal health, concern for the environment, ethical beliefs, and economics. Sometimes it seems there are as many different reasons for changing diets as there are people doing so!

Your reasons are your own, but no matter what your motivation, you will need to embrace the process of change. Before you start actually modifying your diet, I want you to take a moment to think about that process. The time you spend now contemplating the mechanisms of change could make all the difference between success and failure on your path towards vegetarianism.

### It's Just A Habit

Human nature doesn't change, but human customs and habits can and do. Think about all the things people used to do that we no longer do. Think about the clothes our great-great-grandparents wore, the way they traveled, and the work they did. Some people still choose to live that way, but the vast majority of us, no matter how conservative, are living lives that would be unrecognizable to our ancestors. If your great-great-grandparents were to appear on your doorstep tomorrow, they would probably be frightened, or even horrified, by many of the things you now take for granted, from lipstick to automobiles to MTV.

Although customs and habits change, they don't change all at once, nor would we want them to. As humans, we are able to live in many different ways. In order to get along with each other and to have some idea of what to expect of our futures, we have to have some common rules. When cultures clash, as they all too frequently do in our modern world, people become confused. This confusion can lead to a backlash, where people try to recreate the world they thought they knew. But it can also lead to new customs that incorporate the best of the old while discarding the rest.

## Different Diets for Different Folks

The American diet is presently undergoing just such a cultural change. For much of this century, we have been eating what is commonly called the Standard American Diet (SAD), which contains a large proportion of animal products in the form of meat, dairy, and eggs. Over the past several years, however, more and more people have come to question the wisdom of that diet, and have begun to change their own eating habits in consequence.

Not surprisingly, this change in our customs and habits has generated the sort of confusion described above. It may help to step back and view our diets more objectively in order to find our way to a new consensus.

When it comes to food, humans are by nature omnivorous. We can eat anything. We can eat yeasts and fungi and roots and leaves and fruits and grains and nuts and seeds and insects and reptiles and crustaceans and birds and mammals (whew!). At one time or another, in one place or another, humans have eaten grubs and grasshoppers, rats and roaches, cats and cows, and even other humans.

Despite this vast menu, what we eat is largely determined by the society we live in. What we eat is determined not by nature, but by custom and by habit. What we eat can therefore be changed.

That's what this book is all about—changing the foods you eat. In making the decision to become a vegetarian, you are uniting with millions of other people who are striving to come to grips with new knowledge about the effects of diet on our health, the environment, animals, global and personal economy, and much more.

Before you continue, you will need a pen or pencil as well as something to write on. Space has been provided in the following pages, but if you need more room or you don't want to write in the book, I suggest using a separate notebook or a binder filled with lined paper. When you have your writing materials ready, read on!

## Begin at the Beginning

In order to become a vegetarian, you first have to know what one is! The term "vegetarian" is often used loosely in our society, so in the following section I offer a brief outline of the history of vegetarianism followed by an exact definition of the word "vegetarian." This information is intended to help you decide just how you want your diet to evolve.

### An Ancient and Honored Tradition

Throughout history, people from all over the world have eaten a plant-based diet for a variety of reasons. Before the arrival of the European explorers, for example, many agrarian Native American tribes ate a primarily vegetarian diet because plant foods were plentiful and easy to store, and game had become scarce after several hundred years of settlement. Other near-vegetarian tribal cultures include the Vilcabambans (Ecuador), the Abkhasians (former Soviet

Union), and the Hunzas (Himalayas), all of whom are famous for their health and longevity.[1]

In the ancient Western world, great philosophers such as Pythagoras, Plutarch, and Plato advocated a meatless diet for health, aesthetic, and ethical reasons. Similarly, a vegetarian diet has long been an important part of the Hindu and Buddhist religions. Millions of people throughout the world have consequently been, and continue to be, vegetarian.

The word "vegetarian" was coined in England in 1842 by a group of people who promoted a meatless diet for health and ethical reasons. Contrary to popular belief, the word "vegetarian" does not simply mean "vegetable eater." Instead, it was derived from the Latin "homo vegetus" which indicates a healthy and vigorous person.[2] To be a vegetarian is thus to be filled with vitality and life. This usually entails eating some vegetables, but vegetarians are certainly not limited to vegetables alone!

In 1847, the original British Vegetarian Society was formed. Within a short time, the word "vegetarian" had entered the everyday language, and in the years that followed, vegetarianism grew dramatically into a full-fledged social movement.

The growth of vegetarianism slowed during the early part of this century, but both individuals and groups such as the Seventh-day Adventists continued to experiment with the possibilities of a vegetarian diet. When many young people in the 1960s began to question traditional values, vegetarianism gained new prominence. Cuisines from all over the world were rediscovered and combined with more common European and American foods to form the basis of an exciting new diet.

Today, vegetarian cuisine has reached a high level of culinary excellence, and the vegetarian movement is growing rapidly, as more and more people discover its benefits. As many as seven percent of Americans and twelve percent of Britons now consider themselves to be vegetarian.[3,4]

## A Rose By Any Other Name

According to the original Vegetarian Society, a vegetarian is "one who abstains from flesh, fish, and fowl, and who may or may not use milk, eggs, and cheese." Modern variations on this theme are listed below.

*Vegetarian:* A person who does not eat any meat (that is, flesh, meaning: red meat, fowl, fish, and seafood) or meat by-products such as gelatin and lard.

*Lacto-Ovo Vegetarian:* A person who does not eat meat or meat by-products, but who does eat dairy products (lacto) and eggs (ovo).

*Lacto Vegetarian:* A person who does not eat meat or meat by-products or eggs, but who does eat dairy products.

*Ovo Vegetarian:* A person who does not eat meat or meat by-products or dairy products, but who does eat eggs.

*Vegan\* or Dietary Vegan:* A person who does not eat meat, meat by-products, dairy products, or eggs. Many vegans also avoid eating other animal products such as honey.

*Ethical Vegan:* A person who is a strict dietary vegan and who also avoids animal products in non-food items such as clothing (fur, wool, down, silk), household products, cosmetics, medicines, entertainment, etc.

*Omnivore:* Any person who eats both flesh and plants is properly termed an omnivore.

---

\* In my experience, the preferred pronunciation is "VEE-gun." I used to say "VAY-gun," but I stopped when someone said to me, "Vay-guns are from Las Vegas—or perhaps the planet Vega!"

## The Great Debate

Simple though they are, the above definitions are still being debated. One example is honey-avoiding vegans who then don't consider people who eat honey to be vegan even if they don't eat any other animal products. I sometimes joke that there are vegan-A's (who don't eat honey) and vegan-B's (who sometimes do). The debate over such details is ongoing and unlikely to end soon, and it is why I have made a distinction between dietary and ethical veganism. Just keep in mind that it is considered polite to let vegans know whether any items such as honey have been used in preparing food so they can decide if it meets their personal criteria.

The most controversy is raised by the many omnivores who avoid red meat or who eat a primarily, but not completely, vegetarian diet and yet call themselves vegetarians. This practice has made it difficult for true vegetarians when they eat in restaurants or other people's homes. All too often, vegetarians have to fend off offers of fish and chicken, or find themselves eating soup made with chicken broth. Activists also have difficulty advocating vegetarianism because the general public is unclear about what is being discussed.

To help clear up the matter, I offer the following thoughts. Depending on religious proscriptions and cultural beliefs, an omnivore may avoid certain types of flesh. For example, Hindus do not eat cows, Muslims do not eat pigs, and most Americans do not eat cats or dogs or horses. But the avoidance of a particular type of flesh does not a vegetarian make. Therefore, a person who does not eat red meat, but does eat fish or chicken, is not a vegetarian. He is an omnivore who does not eat red meat.

If you are still not convinced, you might consider whether a person who drinks wine, but does not drink hard liquor, could be called a teetotaler. Of course not! To be a teetotaler is to not drink any alcohol. Likewise, to be a vegetarian is to not eat any meat. It really is an either-or proposition.

Some omnivores have attempted to come up with new words such as "pescarian" (fish eater) and "pollarian" (poultry eater), but these ideas have not as yet caught on, probably because eating fish and poultry is still mainstream. As more people change their diets, maybe such distinctions among omnivores will become part of the language. For the sake of clarity, I can only hope so.

Similar comments can be made concerning lacto-ovo vegetarians who describe themselves as vegan. I therefore stick to the above strict definitions and encourage you to do the same. If you are not ready to "go all the way" and avoid flesh altogether, then call yourself an omnivore who eats a plant-based diet (as opposed to an omnivore who eats an animal-centered diet). Similarly, you can be a lacto-ovo vegetarian who eats a near-vegan diet. You can also specify that you want a vegetarian or a vegan meal. But please don't call yourself a vegetarian, or a vegan, until you really are one!

One caveat: the strictest vegetarian will sometimes get slipped a Mickey when eating out. Horror stories abound in vegetarian circles. Also, during the first few months you might "fall off the wagon" once or twice before you get the hang of things. Accidents do happen and are not grounds for not calling yourself a vegetarian. Just learn from your mistakes and vow to be more careful next time.

### What Do You Want To Be?

Now that you know what a vegetarian is, you need to determine what type of vegetarian you want to be. In the following space (or in your notebook), write down your goal. Do you want to be a lacto-ovo vegetarian or a vegan? Or do you really want to remain an omnivore while eating a primarily vegetarian diet? By defining your goal now, you will find the process of change easier and more direct.

*I want to be the following type of vegetarian:*

_____

_____

_____

_____

## Why, Oh Why?

So far, so good! You now know what type of diet you're aiming for. The next step is to explore why you want to make this change.

Why do you need to know why? Because the more focused your reasons, the more likely you are to succeed in changing your diet, and the more likely you are to continue with your new diet in the future. If you understand your motivation, you will be inspired, and the more inspired you are, the easier the change will be.

There are many reasons to become vegetarian, and each person's story is unique. Several common themes have emerged with time, however, and you will probably identify with at least one.

On the pages which follow, I have summarized the most common reasons to become a vegetarian. A few statistics and other details have been included where necessary, but in the interest of brevity, I have kept the descriptions as general as possible. After you have read through them, you will have an opportunity to write down your own thoughts on the subject. If you haven't thought about it before, take your time. The more you understand your own desires, the better.

## Common Reasons to Become a Vegetarian

### — *Health* —

Numerous studies over the past century have made it clear that our present diet is unhealthy, if not downright dangerous. Consumption of large amounts of animal products has been strongly implicated in the so-called "diseases of excess," such as heart attacks, cancer, and stroke—which together account for more than half the deaths in the U.S.

Now the federal government is amending its earlier dietary recommendations. In 1988 C. Everett Koop's first Surgeon General's Report on Nutrition and Health called for more consumption of complex carbohydrates and fiber and reduced intake of fat and cholesterol. The United States

## LEADING CAUSES OF DEATH IN THE U.S.

Diet plays a significant part in contributing to the top three leading causes of death in the United States.

| Rank | Cause of Death | Percent of Total Deaths | Diet-related |
|------|----------------|-------------------------|--------------|
| 1 | Heart Disease | 28.8 | YES |
| 2 | Cancer | 20.5 | YES |
| 3 | Stroke | 5.8 | YES |
| 4 | Chronic lung disease | 3.9 | – |
| 5 | Accidents | 3.5 | – |
| 6 | Pneumonia and influenza | 3.2 | – |
| 7 | Diabetes mellitus | 2.1 | YES |
| 8 | HIV/AIDS | 1.4 | – |
| 9 | Suicide | 1.2 | – |
| 10 | Homicide | 1.0 | – |

*Source:* The National Center for Health Statistics.
Percentages are for the year 1993.

## GOVERNMENT RECOGNITION

At last, the U.S. government—long a supporter of the meat and dairy industries—has a good word for vegetarianism. The 1995 edition of *Nutrition and Your Health: Dietary Guidelines for Americans*, a report first issued in 1980 and updated every five years, contains for the first time the following wording:

"Some Americans eat vegetarian diets for reasons of culture, belief, or health. Most vegetarians eat dairy products and eggs and, as a group, these lacto-ovo vegetarians enjoy excellent health. Vegetarian diets are consistent with the Dietary Guidelines and can meet Recommended Dietary Allowances for nutrients. Protein is not limited in vegetarian diets as long as the variety and amounts of foods consumed are adequate. Meat, fish, and poultry are major contributors of iron, zinc, and B-vitamins in most American diets, and vegetarians should pay special attention to these nutrients.

"Vegans eat only food of plant origin. Because animal products are the only food sources of vitamin $B_{12}$, vegans must supplement their diets with a source of this vitamin. In addition, vegan diets, particularly those of children, require care to assure adequacy of vitamin D and calcium, which most Americans obtain from dairy products."

The Dietary Guidelines are presented by a joint committee of the U.S. Department of Health and Human Services and the U. S. Department of Agriculture. This recognition of vegetarian and vegan diets is one more step in the trend toward official endorsement of healthy alternatives to meat-centered diets.

Department of Agriculture (USDA) followed suit in the early 1990s by replacing the Basic Four Food Groups, which emphasized meat, milk, and eggs, with the Eating Right Pyramid, which emphasizes grains, fruits, and vegetables.

Animal products are much more likely to cause food poisoning than are plants. Salmonella and E. coli bacteria, as well as other pathogenic organisms, are often present in and on animal foods. Cooking destroys some organisms but not others. Food poisoning organisms can also be spread to other foods through the careless handling of animal products. By avoiding animal foods and carefully washing all produce, the risk of food poisoning can be substantially decreased.

Some authorities are now advising that infants not be fed cow's milk because foreign proteins might cause immune system damage that can lead to problems such as juvenile diabetes.[5] Allergies to other foods may also have their root in a childhood allergy to dairy products.

Finally, plant foods are much less likely to contain contaminants that have been linked to various cancers and

---

### BRITISH BEEF

The recent deaths in England from Creutzfeldt-Jakob disease (CJD) have raised questions about the safety of the entire British beef supply. CJD is the human parallel to bovine spongiform encephalopathy, or Mad Cow disease, a fatal disorder in which the victim's brain is destroyed. Eating infected beef is assumed to be the cause of the human deaths, and while hundreds of thousands of British cattle have been killed in an attempt to curb the disease, at this writing, Mad Cow is still a threat to both animals and human. No British beef has legally entered the U.S. for over a decade, but food and cosmetics containing British beef by-products can still be legally imported.

infertility. Animal foods are responsible for 95 to 99 percent of the pesticides and other toxic residues which Americans ingest.[6] Other possible contaminants from animal products are hormone residues which may contribute to premature puberty,[7] and antibiotic residues which can reduce the effectiveness of antibiotic medicines.[8,9]

## — Athletic Performance —

A vegetarian diet has been found to improve fitness as well as health. In consequence, more and more athletes, both amateur and professional, are improving their diets in order to maximize their performance. Preventing cardiovascular problems is of obvious benefit for any athlete. The fittest person in the world can have a heart attack if his arteries are clogged. A low-fat vegetarian diet can also help athletes control their body fat levels and overall weight.

Even more interesting are the numerous studies which have found that a vegetarian diet substantially increases endurance and strength while decreasing recovery time.[10] Olympic track star Carl Lewis, six-time Ironman Triathalon winner Dave Scott, and tennis great Martina Navratilova have all thrived on a vegetarian diet.

## — The Environment —

During the past few decades, it has become increasingly clear that many environmental problems are connected to, if not caused by, the animal agriculture industry. These problems include the deterioration of the ozone layer, the greenhouse effect, groundwater pollution, topsoil loss, deforestation, desertification, drought, pesticide contamination, and species extinction.

This environmental destruction is directly linked to the sheer number of animals necessary to maintain prevailing dietary habits. According to the USDA, over eight billion land animals are killed each year in the United States alone, and that staggering number does not even include certain classes of animals such as the male chicks discarded by the egg industry.[11] And whether they are large like cows or small like chickens, all of those billions of animals, and the breeding herds and flocks from which they come, must have their biological needs met while they are alive. At the end of their lives, they must also be transported, killed, and processed, requiring further use of resources.

Huge tracts of land are used, and abused, by grazing and feed growing operations. Enormous quantities of water irrigate the fields or are contaminated with feces and urine from confinement systems. Metals and plastics are used to build cages and other equipment. Fossil fuels and energy plants run the transport trucks, factory farms, slaughter-houses, and refrigerators. According to a 1978 government study, a full one-third of all raw materials used for all pur-poses in the United States were used in the production of meat, milk, and eggs.[12]

While the livestock industry damages the land, the fish-ing industry damages the sea. According to the United Nations Food and Agriculture Organization, 60 percent of the world's marine stocks are either heavily exploited, fully exploited, or overexploited.[13] The damage done by the fish-ing industry to the oceans, and therefore to the entire envi-ronment of the planet, is incalculable.

*— Animals —*

Discussing vegetarianism without discussing animal agriculture and slaughter is impossible. Our society indulges in a strange kind of mental fog regarding the real-ity of the lives of the animals we eat. We are exposed to numerous documentaries about wolves and whales, but we know next to nothing about the cows, pigs, and chickens who surround us, and quite literally become us.

This is a very emotional subject for many people, and the details may distress you, but I nevertheless urge you to read the following description of the life of a modern dairy cow. Aside from a personal visit to a factory farm or slaughterhouse, reading such descriptions is the best way to gain an understanding of this reason to become a vegetarian.

Dairy calves are separated from their mothers soon after birth. The males are either confined in veal crates, to be killed a few weeks later, or they are castrated and fattened for slaughter in the same manner as beef-type steers. The females, called heifers, are raised to follow their mothers as milk producers.

During her early life, a heifer usually has her ears notched or tagged and any extra teats cut off. She is branded, usually with hot irons, and may also be dehorned. Her development is often speeded with hormones, drugs, and feed supplements. When she begins to ovulate, she is impregnated, usually through artificial insemination. Her pregnancy ends nearly a year later, and her calf is removed soon after.

Deprived of her calf, the cow is milked dry two or three times a day in order to stimulate milk production. Drugs such as Bovine Growth Hormone (BGH) might also be used to increase her production of milk. She may be free to graze in a field between milkings, but more and more dairy cows are being kept in some sort of confinement system. Many of them are chained into narrow stalls for the majority of their lives.

After giving birth, the cow is re-inseminated as soon as possible to ensure future production. The next four to six years of her life are a ceaseless round of milking, pregnancy, birth, and more milking. After that time, she is exhausted and becomes unable to conceive again. Alternatively, she might become injured or diseased. She is then trucked off to the auction yard and ultimately the slaughterhouse.[14,15,16]

On the trucks, the cow may be overheated or exposed to freezing temperatures. Often she is deprived of food, water, and rest. Upon reaching the slaughterhouse, she is prodded down the chutes until she is stunned (if she is lucky) by having a bolt shot into her brain. Her hind leg is then shackled, and she is suspended upside down from a conveyor belt. Death comes from a cut to her throat.[17,18] The lives, and the deaths, of other types of livestock are similar, if not worse.

The animals we eat are not the only ones who suffer. Animals are also experimented upon in laboratories, often (ironically) to find cures for diseases caused by a diet of animal products. In addition, wild animals are hunted, poisoned, and trapped in pest and predator control programs designed to protect feed grains in storage or cows and sheep grazing on public lands. Entire species, including declining populations of songbirds, are pushed to the brink of extinction as habitats are destroyed to create range land and fields of feed grain. And untold billions of organisms die as the fishing industry strips the oceans with its huge trawlers and nets.

### — Humans —

If we rarely talk about the animals we eat, we even more rarely discuss the effects of our modern animal agricultural system on humans.

Because of its inherent wastefulness, animal agriculture has always been the province of the rich. Human beings who are poor are driven off arable lands so that luxury products, such as beef, may be produced for those who can afford them. The result is that people starve to death, or are severely malnourished, in countries which have enough land to feed their populations but instead use this resource to feed livestock.

One tragic example is Ethiopia. At the same time as Americans wept for the starving children with their bloated bellies, the country of Ethiopia was growing and exporting livestock feed grains to the Western world.[19]

Within the borders of the United States, poor people suffer from a similar mal-distribution of food resources as our small farms are swallowed up by large corporations. In addition, the poor are often forced to work in undesirable jobs such as those available on factory farms, in slaughterhouses, or in packing plants, where conditions may be dangerous and unhealthy. Slaughterhouses have some of the highest injury and job turnover rates of any occupation in the nation.[20,21]

Finally, millions of people are crippled and killed by the "diseases of excess" mentioned above. A change in our national diet would greatly improve the health of our friends and families, saving unnecessary tragedy and grief.

### — Personal Economics —

A vegetarian diet can be remarkably inexpensive, especially if highly processed foods are avoided. Grains, legumes, and seasonal produce are cheap and plentiful throughout the United States. People with access to land for a vegetable garden or a small fruit orchard can save even more money.

Another advantage is less need for costly medical care. As discussed above, a vegetarian diet can help prevent many diseases and food poisonings as well as possibly limiting food allergies. Substantial savings on medical insurance, medical bills, and drugs is the inevitable result. You can also work harder and earn more money if you are healthy.

### — Political Protest —

Billions of tax dollars go to subsidizing animal agriculture. Water and energy subsidies, cheap grazing on public lands, predator control programs, price supports, hunting programs, medical and agricultural research grants, meat inspection programs, even military intervention to protect our access to raw materials which are largely used by animal agriculture—all are paid for with our taxes.

For example, calculations have been done to show that plain ground beef would cost around $35 a pound at the cash register if the water used by the cattle industry were not so heavily subsidized.[22] Additional costs may come from the subsidized use of other resources or the need to clean up environmental damage or cover medical expenses. We pay these hidden costs at tax time rather than consciously paying them at the grocery store. Becoming a vegetarian—and letting your elected representatives know why—is an excellent way to protest this expenditure of your tax dollars.

Vegetarianism is also a way to protest the undue influence of Political Action Committees (PACS). According to Common Cause, agribusiness is ranked third in the top ten PAC donors to congressional candidates over the last decade.

Taxpayers are also funding Medicare and other health insurance programs that are then used by people made sick by an animal-centered diet. The health care system is being overwhelmed by our nation's unhealthy lifestyle. A society-wide change to a plant-based diet would help reverse this trend.

## — Aesthetics —

Corpses and raw meat are not beautiful. In a conscious effort to avoid offending their sensibilities, many people in our society refuse to look at meat until it has either been processed or prepared. They also refuse to discuss what goes on at factory farms and slaughterhouses. A butcher shop does not distress them, but a photograph of a slaughterhouse does.

The media assists this societal amnesia through the use of euphemisms and by avoiding images of animals being killed. For example, when was the last time you saw a full-length television documentary on the life of a factory-farmed veal calf or laying hen? How about a full-color magazine photo spread extolling the wonders of working in America's slaughterhouses? Such omissions speak volumes about our culture.

For some people no amount of subterfuge can disguise meat's true nature. Just as most people in the United States recoil at the idea of killing, butchering, and eating the family dog, so have many people stopped eating cows and other animals because they can no longer pretend that what they are eating is not part of a corpse. For these people, the thought of eating meat—any meat—is literally nauseating, and they have ceased to consider meat to be food.*

If the aesthetic argument still fails to move you, you can use your imagination to break through the cultural conditioning that surrounds meat consumption. Three "imagination" exercises follow. If you have never killed and butchered an animal yourself, you will very likely be disturbed by the images you create in your mind. But if you persist, you will have a much greater appreciation of this reason for becoming a vegetarian.

Start by picturing yourself running up to a cow in a field. Imagine throwing yourself onto her neck and biting through to her jugular vein with your teeth or breaking her neck with the weight of your body. In the unlikely event that you killed the cow, rather than vice-versa, imagine then getting down on all fours next to her corpse and, again with just your teeth, attempting to rip through her hide and into her guts the way lions and other carnivores do. Not very appetizing? Exactly!

Another experiment you can try is to look very, very closely at a road-killed animal and imagine scraping the remains off the pavement and eating them right then and there, or even taking them home and cooking them. (Watch out for cars while you do this!) Several joke books have been published on this subject, but actually doing it would be a very different matter for most people.

---

* Recall that "food" is a culturally defined term. In Korea, dogs are food. In the United States, dogs are not food. If enough people cease to consider cows, pigs, chickens, tuna, etc., to be "food," they won't be!

And finally, the next time you are in a butcher's shop, make an attempt to count the number of animals whose bodies are there. In your imagination, put the chickens back together with their hearts, livers, legs, wings, breasts, feathers, and heads. Imagine each chicken is alive and breathing and warm. Focus on one re-united body and imagine it moving around, scratching at the floor, and preening. Continue on to count the cow's tongues—one cow each—and the pig's feet. Each ham is the thigh of a pig and each lamb's leg came off a real lamb. Likewise, all the cuts of beef can be mentally reassembled into a cow. By proceeding in this manner, you will develop a very good feeling for how many animals are killed in this country every day. You can also fill in any mysterious blanks in your knowledge concerning what happens to animals between the field and the kitchen.

### — Evolutionary History/Natural Diet —

Studies of other primates, archeological remains, modern-day "primitive" tribes, and human physiology have made it clear that the bulk of the original human diet consisted primarily of roots, leaves, nuts, seeds, wild grains, and fruits. Our ancestors then probably supplemented this plant-based diet with insects and grubs plus the occasional flesh. During the millions of years before the development of effective tools, red meat was most likely scavenged from corpses left by carnivorous predators. Even after the advent of tool use, flesh probably continued to be a relatively small percentage of the total diet compared to the amounts we eat now.

As for other animal foods, eating eggs would have been a rare, seasonal event, and dairy products would never have been eaten after weaning because of the difficulty of obtaining them from wild animals. For humans in a completely natural state, all foods, including flesh, were of course eaten raw or perhaps dried.[23]

*— Religion/Spirituality —*

Most religions and spiritual traditions call for non-violence and/or concern for animal welfare which is sometimes interpreted as supporting a vegetarian diet. Some religions actively require their members to abstain from animal products.

All of the Judeo-Christian religions, for example, have been influenced by the Old Testament commandment, "Thou shalt not kill." Jewish and Christian vegetarians logically argue that the commandment does not say "Thou shalt not kill humans." They also point to several other passages in the Old Testament which offer further support for their position. A few denominations, such as the Seventh-day Adventists, take this so seriously that a large percentage of their members have become vegetarian.

Some Jews have changed their diets because of the manner in which kosher laws are implemented in modern-day slaughterhouses. Originally designed to minimize the suffering of animals during slaughter, the kosher laws presently cause more suffering for animals because they are not stunned prior to being shackled and hung upside down. In addition to reacting to this inhumane slaughter, many Jews have found that keeping a kosher kitchen is much simpler with a vegetarian diet.

The followers of Hinduism and Buddhism treat vegetarianism much more seriously than do the followers of most Judeo-Christian religions. Hinduism has been greatly influenced by Jainism, which is based on the concept of ahimsa, the principle of least harm. Likewise, the first precept of Buddhism is "refrain from destroying life." Practitioners of both religions therefore hold vegetarianism as an ideal to be encouraged.

The modern Western movement for peace and non-violence that began in the 1960s has been greatly influenced by these Eastern religions. The concept of ahimsa has held special appeal for the peace movement because of its association with Mahatma Gandhi, who was a lacto-vegetarian Hindu.

Members of the feminist and environmental movements have also begun to explore non-violent spirituality through rediscovered Goddess religions and the eco-feminist movement. A plant-centered diet is becoming the norm among these activists as they educate themselves about the violence done to humans (especially women), animals, and the environment by our meat-oriented culture.

## Your Turn

To learn more about any of the above topics, you may want to refer to the Resources chapter of this book, which lists a number of publications that go into detail about the ethics of vegetarianism. If you're not sure why you want to become a vegetarian, you may want to read some of those books before continuing on with this one. The stronger your reasons, and the more reasons you have, the more likely you are to succeed. When you are ready, write down your own thoughts and feelings about becoming a vegetarian. Whatever your reasons, define them as well as you can.

*I want to be a vegetarian because:*

_____

_____

_____

_____

_____

_____

## How Now, Brown Cow

Great! You now know why you want to be a vegetarian as well as what vegetarian diet you are aiming for. You are ready to move on to the fun part—how to actually become one! The Five Step process which follows is designed to help you do just that by leading you easily from your present diet to a vegetarian diet.

A brief synopsis of the Five Step process will give you an idea of the time commitment involved. The process begins with Steps One and Two, which are designed to help you analyze your present diet. The analysis is simple, and will probably take you anywhere from a few hours to a few days, depending on how well acquainted you are with your dietary habits.

In Steps Three and Four you will actively search out and experiment with new foods. Because this necessarily entails spending some time in grocery stores and in the kitchen, these two central steps will require some large chunks of time. You can expect to spend anywhere from several days to several weeks, or even months, on the third and fourth steps depending on your present knowledge of vegetarian foods, your work schedule, and your motivation level.

Step Five is both the simplest and the most demanding. The simple part entails summarizing your work from the other four steps. The demanding part is finalizing your commitment to being a vegetarian. The time commitment for Step Five will be determined, therefore, by how long it takes you to make that final commitment, whether it's one second, one day, one week, or one year. The other four steps will have given you the knowledge you need to be a vegetarian. Step Five is designed to give you the motivation for putting that knowledge to use.

I advise you not to wait too long between steps because your diet will probably change during the course of time anyway, which would send you back to the beginning. You also might lose your motivation if you put off working through the process. On the other hand, it is important not to rush yourself, either. If you are very busy, or hesitant about trying new things, you might need to take a little bit longer in order to avoid overburdening yourself.

If you are made anxious by the changes you are making, then slow down—but don't stop! You'll get there in the end no matter what speed you go. Just remember, you are not alone. Millions of other people are with you on this.

As an additional motivating factor, I have included the idea of "time goals," to help you move through the Five Step process. Start now by deciding how quickly you want to complete all five of the steps. Get out a calendar and choose a date. Be realistic. If you are already aware of your eating habits, have previous experience with vegetarian cooking, and have made a firm commitment to being a vegetarian, the entire process could take as little as a week or a month. If, on the other hand, you have never before analyzed your diet, have never knowingly cooked a vegetarian meal, and are still not sure of the strength of your commitment, the process could take considerably longer, perhaps as long as six months or a year.

Choose a date which will allow you plenty of leeway, but not so much that you lose your inspiration. I suggest that you choose to finish the entire Five Step process sometime between four and six months after you start. That should give you plenty of time to try new foods without feeling pressured while at the same time motivating you to complete the process. And if you finish sooner than that, think how good you will feel!

*I plan to finish the entire Five Step process by:*

_____

You will be given opportunities to choose secondary time goals for the completion of the individual steps as you proceed through the process. In that way, you will work your way through the process by your target date.

If you are unable to complete one of the steps in the time you set, don't feel bad; just go back and reschedule. Having a time-frame firmly in mind can help you overcome any tendency to procrastinate. Also, if you find yourself continually putting off a step, you may have fears or uncertainties that need to be addressed. In the Resources chapter, you will find the titles of some books on the psychology of change that can help you overcome any difficulties you encounter.

When you are ready, move on to Step One!

# The
# Five Steps

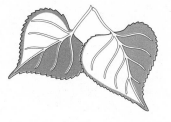

# Step One:
## What You Eat Now

In order to change any habit you need to know what you are doing now. The first step in the Five Step process, therefore, is to analyze your present everyday eating habits by making a list of the foods you currently eat. When this step is complete, you will know exactly where you are and will be in a position to move towards something else. This step is essential to the success of the program, so take as long as you need, whether a few hours or a few days. The more thoroughly you analyze your present diet, the easier the other steps, and your change to a new way of eating, will be.

The best way to learn is through example, so I have provided one which will accompany you as you proceed through the steps. By carefully studying the example before you do each step for yourself, you will gain the confidence you need to proceed on your own. Any time you get stuck, just go back and look at the example for that section again. It may be all you need to give you that added boost over a difficult spot.

On the next page, you'll find the example for Step One. It is a list of foods similar to those that might be regularly eaten by a hypothetical, non-vegetarian "average American." I've kept it fairly short and simple; your own list will probably be somewhat longer. Take a moment to go through the list. It will be used throughout the book, so you'll want to be familiar with it right from the start.

## STEP ONE *Example:*
## *What I Eat Now*

Cereal with milk

Doughnuts or pastries

Orange juice

Coffee with cream

Scrambled eggs with bacon

Toast with jam

Roast beef or turkey sandwich (deli)

Potato salad (deli)

Chicken chow mein

Pepperoni and mushroom pizza

Soft drinks

Apples

Carrot sticks

Cheese on crackers

White wine

Split pea soup (contains pork) with French Bread

Meatloaf

Macaroni and cheese

Tuna salad sandwich

Baked potato with butter

Mixed green salad with ranch dressing

Beef and cheese tacos

Corn chips with salsa or bean dip

Shrimp and vegetable stir-fry over rice

Ice cream

Cookies

Lasagna with meat sauce (Birthday dinner)

Cheeseburger

Bananas

Broccoli

Pancakes

Tomato slices

## Green Eggs and Ham

You'll notice in the example that some foods are listed together rather than separately. If you always eat bacon with your eggs, or always have cream in your coffee, it doesn't make sense to put the different elements on different lines. Actually, it is part of the education process to note which foods you usually eat in combination with others.

Also observe that ingredients of processed and prepared foods are not listed separately. Instead, foods are listed as they are eaten. For example, if you eat raw apples then you will obviously put down "apples." If you eat apple pie you would not put down apples, but would instead list "apple pie."

One exception to that rule occurs when a food has a known animal product "hidden"in it, such as the pork in the split pea soup. You needn't worry about every little nit-picky detail, though. It's enough for now to get the obvious meat and meat products listed. If you miss some obscure ingredient, you can go back and deal with it later.

At the beginning, stick to the foods you eat on a regular basis. Going back to the example, note that the lasagna is a once-a-year birthday dinner and so could be left off the list. After you have become comfortable with your new diet, you can then work on changing your own rarely eaten "special occasion" foods. I've included a section near the end of the book for that very purpose.

## A Journey of a Thousand Miles Starts With the First Step

In the pages ahead, there is a space provided for you to write in, labeled Step One: What I Eat Now. If you are using a separate notebook, label a fresh sheet accordingly. What you are going to do is list your own commonly eaten foods. Keep in mind that this isn't a test, so there are no right or wrong answers!

In this first step—and with all five of the steps—take your time, and be sure to reward yourself when you finish,

## THERE COULD BE COW IN THAT CANDY

If we accept the modern-day homily that we "are what we eat," then we really should know what we eat. This book will help you to know the facts about what's really in some foods that seem innocuous or even entertaining. Beef gelatin, rendered from the hides and bones of cattle, for instance, is an ingredient in most marshmallows and gummy candies. Gelatin is also used in many brands of yogurt, puddings, and baby food. The prevalence of animal-origin ingredients is addressed elsewhere in this book, and a detailed list of these "hidden" substances can be found in the Resources chapter. As you compile your list of commonly-eaten foods, however, you may find it useful to note the snack foods or treats you enjoy—because later you may want to find all-vegetarian substitutes.

because during this process of change, it is very important for you to relieve any stress or anxiety you might be experiencing. After all, this is supposed to be a fun adventure! Make it so by celebrating the successful completion of each step before you move on to the next.

Before you actually begin, take a moment to decide the total amount of time you want to devote to this step. While it is important to have a reasonably accurate and detailed list, it is also important not to get stuck trying to pin down every last little thing you eat. If you forget something, you can always go back and add it in later. After all, if it's really something you eat regularly, you will probably eat it within the next several days, at which time you can write it down.

*I plan to finish Step One by:*

## STEP ONE:
### *What I Eat Now*

# Step Two:
## Categorizing Your Diet

You have completed Step One and now you have a list of foods that you commonly eat. In Step Two, you are going to take that list of foods and break it up into the three major categories we identified in the first section: non-vegetarian, lacto-ovo vegetarian, and vegan.

Earlier I told you not to worry about every last detail, that it is enough to get the obvious animal products out of your diet first. The question is, which are the obvious ones? Just to make sure you know, I am going to list the most common animal ingredients (other than the obvious flesh products, such as pork) that you should be aware of and look for in your own foods. A more complete list is available in the Resources chapter, but I advise you to start with this one.

### Common Animal Ingredients
*Egg products*
Egg whites (albumen)
Egg yolks
Whole eggs
Powdered eggs
*Dairy products*
Milk or milk powder
Whey or whey powder
Cream or whipped cream
Half-and-half
Butter
Casein

*Meat products*
    Rennet
    Gelatin
    Lard
    Animal shortening
    Chicken or beef broth or stock

## Questions, Questions

In many cases it will be fairly clear what the ingredients in your foods are, especially if you prepare your own meals. But if someone else does the cooking or you use a lot of prepared foods, you might have to ask some questions or read some labels. Since this type of investigation is an indispensable part of the program, I want to take a moment to discuss how to go about it.

Learning how to ask questions without antagonizing people is an important part of being a vegetarian in a meat-eating world. First of all, don't be shy about asking questions. You need to know this information, and there is nothing odd or rude in a request about ingredients. Many people are concerned about the effect on their health of animal products, preservatives, chemicals, and various other ingredients. Some people are so chemically sensitive or allergic that asking about ingredients can be a life or death matter. You have a right to seek out this information.

You will probably find that most people are happy to answer your questions, but others are quick to take offense even when no insult is intended. The trick is to frame your queries so as not to challenge other people's beliefs or diet. If someone you question becomes upset, reassure them. Let them know you merely want this information for your own personal use. If they continue to be upset, then don't persist. Find some other way to get the information you need.

## Labels

Another skill you will need is that of reading the list of food ingredients on the labels of processed foods. Since you

## RENNET AND CASEIN

Rennet and casein are the bugaboos of the vegetarian world, and deserve a separate discussion. Rennet is a substance taken from the lining of calves' stomachs which is then used to coagulate cow's milk into cheese. Casein is a protein derived from cow's milk that is used to make soy cheeses melt.

There are some cow's milk cheeses which are made with no rennet or with a plant-based rennet. There are also a few soy cheeses which do not contain any casein. It remains true, however, that most cow's milk cheeses are not strictly vegetarian and most soy cheeses are not strictly vegan.

Since cheese is often a major component of the diets of new vegetarians, I want you to be aware of the presence of rennet and casein, but I don't want you to get hung up on them either. This is one of those gray areas that most vegetarians choose to ignore, at least when eating outside their own homes. So even though I have put them in the above list of common animal ingredients, I advise you to just go ahead and eat your cheese. Later on, you can look into the issue more thoroughly if you decide you want to be more strict.

are going to be doing a lot of label-reading in the future, it pays to familiarize yourself with the rules that govern the listing of food ingredients.

The Food and Drug Administration (FDA) oversees the labeling of most foods, but the United States Department of Agriculture (USDA) has jurisdiction over meats, dairy, and eggs as well as certain foods prepared using those animal products. Fortunately, most labels follow the FDA rules.

When you pick up a prepared food item, you will usually find the list of ingredients in small print near the bottom of the can or on the side of the package. The ingredients are listed in order of amount. In other words, the first ingredient listed is the one present in the greatest amount and on down the line to the last ingredient which is found in the smallest amount.

As a vegetarian, you need to be aware that there are some additives and processes used in preparing certain foods which are not required to be listed on the label. For example, until recent action by religious groups, tin cans were manufactured using animal fats. Another, more distressing example is white sugar, which is bleached through a charcoal made of animal bones. I don't want you to worry about this too much right now; I just want you to be aware of it. For the present, it's enough to know that all of the common animal ingredients I mentioned above (except rennet) will show up on the label if they are present in the food.

## Vegan, Lacto-ovo, or Non-Vegetarian?

Now that you know how to get the information you need, you are ready to learn how to categorize your diet. This is an important step because it will help you get into the swing of understanding the distinctions among vegetarian and non-vegetarian foods. You will soon see, for instance, that vegan foods—thought by some to be just "too weird"— are already a part of your diet. Far from being weird, vegan foods (marinated mushrooms, perhaps, or pita bread, guacamole, no-fat corn chips and salsa, baked potato with broccoli) may be among your very favorites.

To start on your list, first look over the example for Step Two. As you can see, each food from the sample list from Step One has been put into one of the three categories. Some of the foods are vegan (they contain no animal products), some are lacto-ovo vegetarian (they contain milk and/or eggs), and the rest are non-vegetarian (they contain meat or meat by-products). More details about ingredients are noted where appropriate.

**STEP TWO** *Example:*

## Categorizing My Present Diet

### *VEGAN FOODS*

Orange juice

Soft drinks

Apples

Carrot sticks

Crackers (brands which are dairy-free)

White wine

French bread

Corn chips with salsa or bean dip (no lard)

Rice

Bananas

Broccoli

Tomato slices

**STEP TWO** *Example:*

## Categorizing My Present Diet

### LACTO-OVO VEGETARIAN FOODS

Cereal with milk

Doughnuts or pastries (eggs and/or dairy)

Coffee with cream

Scrambled eggs (butter and milk)

Toast with jam (bread contains whey)

Potato salad (mayonnaise has eggs)

Cheese on crackers (contain dairy)

Baked potato with butter

Macaroni and cheese

Mixed green salad with ranch dressing (dairy)

Ice cream

Cookies (eggs and dairy)

Pancakes (eggs)

**STEP TWO** *Example:*

## Categorizing My Present Diet

### NON-VEGETARIAN FOODS

Bacon

Roast beef or turkey sandwich

Chicken chow mein

Pepperoni and mushroom pizza

Split pea soup (contains pork)

Meatloaf

Tuna salad sandwich

Beef and cheese tacos

Shrimp and vegetable stir-fry

Cheeseburger

## Separating the Wheat from the Chaff

Now it's your turn to identify what you currently eat as either vegan, lacto-ovo vegetarian, or non-vegetarian. To do this, you will need your list from Step One. One food at a time, list each item in the appropriate category. You may use the space provided on the next few pages, or use your notebook, if that feels more comfortable. Plant foods will go into the vegan category, foods with dairy and egg products into the lacto-ovo category, and all foods with meat, or obvious meat by-products will go into the non-vegetarian category.

Some items can be split up, like the scrambled eggs and bacon in the example. But if you absolutely have to have butter with your potatoes or cream with your coffee, go ahead and keep them together in this step.

Before you begin, decide how long you want to spend on this task and write your time goal in the space below.

*I plan to finish Step Two by:*

---

### WHATCHA DOIN'?

Your first encounter with anti-vegetarian sentiment may occur when family members or friends observe you making lists of foods and referring frequently to this book. Ways to deal with others who are concerned about your health or who may feel threatened by your goal are covered in the Social Interactions section of chapter four. I encourage you to read those pages if other's comments become distracting. In the meantime, you may want to seek support from a vegetarian friend or acquaintance who will encourage and congratulate you on your efforts.

**STEP TWO:**
*Categorizing My Present Diet*

### *VEGAN FOODS*

**STEP TWO:**
*Categorizing My Present Diet*

### LACTO-OVO VEGETARIAN FOODS

## STEP TWO:
## *Categorizing My Present Diet*

### *NON-VEGETARIAN FOODS*

## Where's the Beef?

Take a moment to study your lists. Are you surprised by the number of items in the first two vegetarian categories? If so, you aren't alone. In our meat-centered society it is easy to forget that the human diet has been and continues to be largely vegetarian. By separating your diet into these categories, you begin to see how distorted our collective image of our diet has become.

Even in the non-vegetarian food category, the dishes often contain a large proportion of plants as well as eggs and dairy products. Consider, for instance, the pizza in the example. Sure, it has pepperoni. But it also has mushrooms and tomato sauce and cheese and a wheat-flour crust. Or how about the split pea soup? It's filled with peas and vegetables while the quarter-sized piece of pork looks like it was added almost as an afterthought.

In many dishes, meat is an add-in, an extra ingredient thought to be necessary for flavor or to make a meal seem "complete." Sometimes we may be eating meat-containing foods out of habit, not recognizing that their vegetarian versions are in fact more palatable. For instance, the bits of beef in vegetable-beef soup may be no more than tough shreds barely recognizable as any kind of food.

We also sometimes add meat or cheese to dishes we make at home or order in restaurants. Chili without beef is quite delicious, however, as is a Greek salad without feta cheese. Your list may include dishes that would be completely vegetarian except for one ingredient!

With your new understanding, continue to look over your own lists before moving on to the next step. Reward yourself for your effort by glorying in all the lacto-ovo vegetarian and vegan foods you already eat. If you are like most people, even if you stopped eating meat tomorrow you would still be able to choose from plenty of foods that you know and like. This alone should reassure you that changing your diet is not only possible, but painless!

# Step Three:
## Rethinking the Categories

Now it's time to really get to work. In Step Three you are going to look for "substitutes" for foods you already eat and like. By substitutes, I mean foods that are similar in taste, texture, and method of preparation to the non-vegetarian foods you are eating now. If you wish to become vegan, you will also look for substitutes for your lacto-ovo foods.

Don't rush yourself. Be patient with your progress, and if you need reassurance, just go back to Step Two and look at all the vegetarian foods you eat already.

In some cases, you'll be able to find a vegetarian substitute easily. In other cases, the search will be more difficult. No matter what the outcome, the idea is to give a good share of the many interesting products on the market the old college try. "Try it, you just might like it," is the name of the game!

### Yes, Tofu is Food

Look at the example for Step Three. Using the lacto-ovo list from Step Two, I have suggested a possible vegan substitute for several of the items. Similarly, I have listed possible vegan (V) or lacto-ovo (LO) substitutes for some of the non-vegetarian foods. It is actually possible to find a lacto-ovo or vegan substitute for every single one of the non-vegetarian items on the original list, and a vegan substitute for every item in the lacto-ovo category. Because finding substitutes can be time-consuming, I have only noted some of the simpler possibilities.

Don't worry if you have never heard of some of these foods or if they sound unappetizing to you. I just want to give you an idea of what is possible. No one is going to force you to eat foods you don't like! But try not to dismiss new foods just because they are new. Maybe you'll like them, maybe you won't, but you can't know until you try!

### Fee, Fie, Faux, Fum

Many people become incensed by the idea of eating "fake" meats. Since there are so many wonderful vegetarian foods found under the heading "fake," this is a good place to discuss the issue.

What is meat? To put it bluntly, meat is muscle tissue and other organs taken from the corpse of an animal. It has a "meaty" texture and is filled with the blood, lymph, urea, and other body fluids that are euphemistically termed "juice."

Before meat is eaten, it is usually processed in some way. Sushi and steak tartare are the rare (pun not intended) exceptions, and even they are presented in a somewhat "processed" fashion. After being processed, meat is no longer just meat. The meat is merely the raw material that was used to make the processed food.

Why not make similar processed foods using different raw materials? A hot dog, for example, is a highly processed food. Originally, hot dogs were made with beef. Several years ago, they began to be made with chicken meat and turkey meat. More recently, they have been made with soybeans. But no matter which way you slice it, they are all hot dogs!

A non-food example might serve to make this more clear. For the last one hundred years or so, paper has been primarily made from wood pulp. Paper, however, can be made from many other materials such as hemp, cotton rags, and sugar cane. Are these papers "fake" because they aren't made from trees? Of course not. And a hot dog made with soybeans is not a "fake" hot dog. So don't feel that you are being some kind of hypocrite by eating vegetarian processed foods that are similar to non-vegetarian processed foods in taste or texture or looks or name.

An important corollary to this is that you must not expect vegetarian versions of certain foods to taste exactly the same as the meat versions (or vegan to taste like lacto-ovo). Sometimes they are very similar, as with hot dogs. Other times they are very different, as with many veggie burgers. If you keep this fact firmly in mind, you will be more open to trying these new foods and less likely to be disappointed.

## HIDE AND SEEK

How far you go to get animal products out of your diet is up to you. You might be satisfied with just getting the obvious meat products out. Or you might find yourself going back again and again to Step Two to revaluate your diet with reference to all the "hidden" animal ingredients which lie in wait for the unwary vegetarian.

In the latter case, you must always keep in mind that perfection is impossible. There will always be the insects in the grain, and you will probably not know if blood meal was used to fertilize the organic fruit, or be aware of the little-known manufacturing process which uses some obscure animal-derived ingredient for which no substitute has (yet!) been found. But given that this is an imperfect world, it is still good to have at least a vision of perfection.

In the Resources chapter of this book, I have compiled a detailed list of animal products that you may find in your food. Many items can come from either plant or animal sources. Which is used usually depends on what is most economical for the manufacturers, so you will have to contact them directly to find out. The list is, of course, not comprehensive. Nor does it include animal products that are used for purposes other than food. To learn more about animal products in cosmetics, clothes, and so on, you need to contact a vegan or animal rights group.

**STEP THREE** *Example:*
## Rethinking the Categories

### VEGAN SUBSTITUTES
### FOR MY LACTO-OVO VEGETARIAN FOODS

| | |
|---|---|
| Cereal with cow's milk | Cereal with soy milk |
| Doughnuts or pastries | |
| Coffee with cream | |
| Scrambled eggs | Scrambled tofu |
| Toast (whey) with jam | Toast (no whey) with jam |
| Potato salad (egg mayo) | |
| Cheese on crackers | Crackers (dairy-free) |
| Baked potato with butter | Baked potato with margarine |
| Green salad w/ranch dressing | Green salad with oil dressing |
| Ice cream | |
| Cookies (eggs and dairy) | Cookies (no eggs or dairy) |
| Pancakes (eggs) | Pancakes (no eggs) |

## STEP THREE *Example:*
## Rethinking the Categories

### VEGETARIAN SUBSTITUTES
### FOR MY NON-VEGETARIAN FOODS

| | |
|---|---|
| Bacon | |
| Roast beef sandwich | |
| Chicken chow mein | Vegetable chow mein (V) |
| Pepperoni pizza | Olive/mushroom pizza (LO) |
| Split pea soup (with pork) | Split pea soup (no pork) (V) |
| Meatloaf | |
| Beef and cheese tacos | Bean and cheese tacos (LO) |
| Shrimp/vegetable stir-fry | Vegetable stir-fry (V) |

## Instituting the Search

In your own search for vegetarian substitutes you could use two techniques. The first is a thorough exploration for simple substitutes at your grocery store, and perhaps some specialty stores as well. The second is the art of modifying recipes.

There will, of course, be some overlap between these two substitution techniques especially for recipes that call for prepared foods. For example, if you have a homemade soup recipe that calls for canned chicken broth, you could substitute canned vegetable broth, a simple miso-and-water broth, or tomato juice.

In addition to spending time at the store, you will need to spend time in the kitchen actively experimenting. How long you spend at both activities will depend on your previous cooking experience as well as how enthusiastic you are about finding substitutes.

If you are an inexperienced cook, keep it simple! Substituting canned vegetable broth for canned chicken broth shouldn't be a problem for anyone, but making scrambled tofu when you have never even made scrambled eggs could be an exercise in frustration until you have gained more experience. This doesn't mean you can't make scrambled tofu if you really want to, but if you aren't ready to attempt it yet, then don't!

In other words, if you find yourself spending an inordinate amount of effort on a particular item, just move on to the next one. It's more important for you not to frustrate yourself than it is to find a substitute for every last thing you now eat. Either you will find substitutes for the more difficult items later (perhaps when doing the next step or perhaps after you have completed the entire process), or you will drop those foods from your diet altogether in favor of other things.

Keeping that in mind, decide now how long you want to spend on Step Three.

*I plan to finish Step Three by:*

_____

### Hi Ho! Hi Ho! It's Off to the Store We Go!

To get started on your search for possible substitutes, you're going to need to get out of the house. The most comfortable place to go is to your usual food store or stores. I would suggest that this first trip not be a shopping trip. Give yourself plenty of time, and go alone so you won't feel rushed or flustered. Be sure to take your list of foods from Step Two. You are specifically looking for simple substitutes for those non-vegetarian or lacto-ovo items that you wish to change. When you find one, write it down. My advice is that you not buy anything yet. Just note where it is for future reference.

I encourage you to write down all the possibilities you encounter whether they look appetizing to you or not. This is an investigation. You don't have to try anything you think looks "yucky," but it is nice to know it's out there in case you change your mind.

The easiest way to proceed is to start at one end of the store and work your way through, keeping an eye out for any item that could be a substitute for an item on your list. Alternatively, you could start at the top of your list and work down through the items one at a time. That will probably entail more walking, but you will be sure not to miss anything. If you can't find what you want, don't be shy about asking for help. The store personnel know their stock and can save you a lot of time. They also might be willing to order an item they don't normally carry.

This trip is not meant to be comprehensive so limit your search to the prepared food items on your list. For example, if you eat a brand of split pea soup that contains pork, then you will want to look in the soup section for a brand of split pea soup that does not contain pork. Once you have found what you want (or have determined that nothing appropriate is available), move on to the next aisle or the next item on your list, depending on your method. Leave the investigation of all the other types of soup for another day.

And again, don't worry if you don't find a substitute for everything on your list. Just do the best you can, and the rest will come with time.

## Let Your Fingers Do the Walking

After you have found all the possible substitutes that are available in your regular store, you might want to look elsewhere. How far you have to go will largely depend on how progressive your shopkeeper is and how determined you are to find substitutes. Some major supermarkets carry an astonishing variety of vegetarian foods; others are in the Dark Ages. If you suspect you are shopping at one of the less enlightened markets, you might want to investigate alternative stores in your area.

.Get out the Yellow Pages, and look up "Foods" or "Supermarkets." Write down the address and hours of any place that looks interesting or different. I suggest you look for specialty markets. For example, there are stores which specialize in ethnic foods such as Indian, Asian, and Middle Eastern. Other stores concentrate on one category of food such as cheese or produce or baked goods.

Next, look up "Health Foods." Avoid the ones that sell mainly vitamins unless they also carry a decent selection of processed and prepared vegetarian foods. The best natural food stores carry lots of high-quality produce, bulk grains, and the like.

As long as you're at it, you might also look to see if there is a vegetarian society listed for your area. They will tell you what stores are available, and can give you advice on finding substitutes. I have also listed some good mail order companies in the Resources chapter. If you live in a rural area, they can be indispensable.

When your list is together, head out the door again! Go through these new stores in exactly the same way that you went through your regular store—with an eye out for substitutes for foods on your list. Don't look at every last thing. There will be plenty of time for that later!

### Try It, You'll Like It (Maybe)

Now that you have an idea of what substitutes are available in the stores, it's time for you to actually try some of them. Go back to the stores with a shopping list and buy several of the items you want to try. When you get home, give them a go!

To increase the chances of success, prepare and serve the substitutes in the same way as your old foods whenever possible. For example, if you always serve your beef burgers on toasted white buns with lots of mustard, ketchup, onions, tomatoes, and pickles along with a side of French fries, be sure to do the same with your veggie burgers. That will ensure a familiar taste which you already know you like.

Don't worry if you don't like something right away. It takes time to learn to enjoy new foods. Remember low-fat milk? Back in the '50s and '60s, everyone drank whole milk. Then we started hearing about how unhealthy it was, so we switched to low-fat and non-fat varieties. Yuck! Low-fat milk was bland and watery and kind of blue-looking. But a funny thing happened. After a while, we started to like it, and the whole milk began to look thick and gloppy. Our tastes had changed.

Another example is whole wheat bread. We thought it was dry and tasteless. Now it's white bread that we characterize as fluffy and bland while stuffing down a huge variety of whole grain breads with gusto.

Give yourself time for your tastes to change. If you absolutely hate one of the substitutes you try—well, maybe it isn't for you. But if it's at all okay, you might give it another chance (or two or three) before making a final decision. And, of course, there will be things you like, or even love, right away. You just have to try them with an open mind in order to find that out.

This is an ongoing process. One of the most exciting things about being a vegetarian these days is all the great new products that are coming out on the market. Keep your eyes open and your taste buds primed. The next thing you try just might be a winner! When it is, write it on the pages for Step Three.

### Modifying Recipes

Finding substitutes for foods you prepare yourself is the next task. As with prepackaged foods, in some cases you will find a substitute you like, in others you won't. With time and experience your success rate will increase, and you will very likely be pleasantly surprised at how sophisticated many vegetarian recipes have become.

The first thing you can do to modify your own recipes is to look in vegetarian cookbooks for recipes that are similar to yours. If you don't have any vegetarian cookbooks, you will need to get some. You might be able to borrow them from the library or from friends, but in the long run, you will be happier if you actually buy them.

The usual advice is to start with three good cookbooks—one basic lacto-ovo, one basic vegan, and one gourmet or specialty. Several good cookbooks have been listed in the Resources chapter, but if you have limited means, I suggest you start with the three cookbooks in the "All-Stars" list. They can be obtained through mail-order or through your local bookstore.

To illustrate how you are going to use your vegetarian cookbooks, let's look at the meatloaf in the original example. In order to find a substitute for meatloaf, you could look up several recipes for nutloafs, grainloafs, beanloafs, tofuloafs, and TVPloafs (TVP stands for textured vegetable protein, a popular substitute for ground beef). You could then prepare several of those recipes until you discover at least one you like.

The second possible modification is a substitution of ingredients in your own recipe. Often this is a simple process. As mentioned before, it is easy enough to use vegetable broth in the place of chicken broth when making soup, although you may have to experiment a bit to find a vegetable broth you like.

When making substitutions in more elaborate recipes, and especially when baking, extra care must be taken. The most experienced of cooks can have some spectacular disasters fiddling around with recipes! To use the previous example, you could replace the hamburger in your old favorite meatloaf recipe with TVP. It might work just fine, but then again, it might not. The advantage of using recipes from cookbooks is that they are pretty sure to come out.

I have listed some of the most common recipe substitutions below. A complete description of how to make these modifications is beyond the scope of this book. For details, look in vegetarian cookbooks and magazines, contact a vegetarian organization, or take a vegetarian cooking class. Keep in mind that the substitutes suggested here are not necessarily nutritionally equal to the items they are replacing. The point I am making is that by modifying your favorite foods—often by just replacing one ingredient—you can transform them to vegan or vegetarian fare.

## Common Substitutes for Animal Ingredients
*Eggs*
*In baking and cooking:*
   Tofu, both regular and silken
*In baking:*
   Ener-G Egg Replacer ®
   Liquid soy lecithin

Flax seeds thoroughly blended in water
Arrowroot powder
Cornstarch
Baking soda (sometimes with vinegar)
Baking powder
Mashed potatoes or squash
Fruit purees

*Cow's milk or goat's milk*
Soy milks (several brands)
Rice milks (several brands)
Nut milks (a few brands or homemade)
Banana milk (homemade)
Fruit and vegetable juices

*Cow's milk or goat's milk cheeses*
Soy cheeses (usually contain casein)
Nut-based cheeses
Nutritional yeast (not brewer's yeast!)

*Cow's milk yogurt, sour cream, whipped cream*
Tofu yogurt, tofu sour cream, whipped tofu

*Butter*
Vegetable shortening
Soy margarine
Vegetable oil
Nut butters
Avocado

*Cow's milk ice cream*
Tofu ice cream
Rice ice cream
Frozen fruit puree

*Meat*
Eggs
Cheese
Tofu and tempeh products
Wheat gluten (seitan)
Textured vegetable protein (TVP)

*Meat Flavor*
Roasted vegetables
Toasted nuts and seeds
Browned onions
Sea vegetables
Miso
Liquid hickory smoke

*Meat broth*
Vegetable broth
Vegetable juices
Miso broth
Bean or lentil broth
Mushroom soaking water
Wine or beer

*Lard*
Butter
Vegetable shortening
Soy margarine
Vegetable oil

*Gelatin*
Tapioca
Agar-agar
Kudzu
Arrowroot powder
Cornstarch

## Halfway to Heaven

After this step, you will have finished well over half of your journey. Your list of vegetarian foods is growing apace and your goal of becoming a vegetarian is fast becoming a reality. Step Three is a major part of the Five Step process, and you can feel proud when you complete it. Before moving on to the next step, be sure to reward yourself appropriately for your accomplishment!

## STEP THREE
*Rethinking the Categories*

### VEGAN SUBSTITUTES
### FOR MY LACTO-OVO VEGETARIAN FOODS

_____     _____

_____     _____

_____     _____

_____     _____

_____     _____

_____     _____

_____     _____

_____     _____

_____     _____

_____     _____

_____     _____

_____     _____

_____     _____

_____     _____

_____     _____

_____     _____

_____     _____

_____     _____

_____     _____

## STEP THREE
# Rethinking the Categories

### VEGETARIAN SUBSTITUTES
### FOR MY NON-VEGETARIAN FOODS

# Step Four:
## Adding New Foods

In the last section, you found substitutes for foods you already know and like. Some of those substitutes were probably pretty tame, such as switching brands of split pea soup. Others undoubtedly took a bit more courage, such as trying a veggie burger for the very first time. Well, prepare to challenge yourself even more! In Step Four, you will be trying all new and different things.

This isn't really any different from what you have been doing all your life. Most people, even the most die-hard omnivores, occasionally try new foods and new recipes. Think of this step as a continuation of that quest, only this time all the new foods and recipes will be vegetarian. Instead of trying venison pie and tripe stew and shark fillets, you will be trying wild mushroom pie and garbanzo bean stew and tempeh fillets. You will experiment with Asian pears and Jerusalem artichokes, barbecued vegetables and cold apple soup, tofu stir-fries and lentil curries.

How many items end up on your list of new vegetarian foods will depend on how adventurous you are, how varied you like your diet to be, and how quickly you want to move through the Five Steps. Some people are happy eating the same few things day after day, while others enjoy making a new gourmet creation every night. To encourage you to try enough foods to complete the Five Steps successfully, I urge you to find at least ten completely new and different foods and recipes that you like and will regularly buy or make.

Please realize that you don't have to become a gourmet cook in order to meet this goal. Vegetarian recipes can be as simple or elaborate as non-vegetarian recipes. If you aren't interested in spending lots of time in the kitchen, emphasize prepared meals from the grocery store and very simple cooked meals such as soup and bread. On the other hand, if you're a cooking fiend, you'll love the challenge of all the new ideas you'll find.

For Step Four, I have written down ten popular vegan foods and ten popular lacto-ovo vegetarian foods. I have included pre-packaged foods, recipes which are very simple to make, and other recipes which require more elaborate preparation. The examples include breakfast, lunch, and dinner items, as well as snacks and desserts. As you search for new foods, you should aim for a similar variety.

## Searching for Ten Good Foods

To complete Step Four you will have to make at least one more long research trip to the grocery store, and you will have to spend some more time in the kitchen. The search for ten new vegetarian foods can take as little as three or four days if you try, and like, something new at each meal. But if you make something new only once a week and you like only every third thing you try, it will take you proportionately longer.

Since preparing and sampling completely unfamiliar foods can be stressful, you might want to schedule special times for your trial meals. Some people find that they like to make a habit of cooking something new at dinner every night or on the weekends. Depending on how quickly you want to complete Step Four, designate one, two, or more days during the week for "adventure" meals. The date you picked for finishing the entire Five Step process will help you decide how long, and how often, you want to experiment with new foods before proceeding to the next, and final, step.

*I plan to finish Step Four by:*

**STEP FOUR** *Example:*
## My New Vegan Foods

Soy milk French toast with maple syrup

Veggie burger with "the works"

Falafel-tahini sandwich (deli)

Jicama

Sesame seed breadsticks

Tofu and broccoli stir-fry over millet

Lentil dahl with potatoes

Portobello mushrooms, marinated and grilled

Steamed greens (e.g., swiss chard, collards)

Fruit crumble

**STEP FOUR** *Example:*
## My New Lacto-Ovo Vegetarian Foods

Oatmeal with banana, walnuts, cow's milk

Soy sausages (egg whites)

Spanish omelette

Roasted red pepper and cheese sandwich (deli)

Spinach cheese puffs

Cream of broccoli soup

Polenta with creamy mushroom gravy

Vegetable pot pie (cow's milk)

Egg pasta with marinara sauce, Parmesan cheese

Cheesecake

## Just Take it One Aisle at a Time

Put on your walking shoes because it's time for another, more detailed "look-see" trip to your grocery store. When you did Step Three, I asked you to limit yourself to looking for specific substitutes for foods you already eat. Now, you are going to roam the aisles keeping an eye out for completely new foods and products that you have probably never noticed before. If you shop at a very large store, this could take a few hours, so make sure you're well rested and raring to go!

As you go through the store, don't buy anything, but note the name and location of whatever you think looks interesting. By the end of the trip, you should have lots of ideas for adventurous future meals.

Start in the produce section. Have you really looked at all the fruits and vegetables that are being offered these days? Most people just head straight for the same old carrots and apples and iceberg lettuce. This time, start on one side and go to the other, looking at everything along the way. Pick up that unusual root and weigh it in your hand. Examine that weird vegetable and the strange new fruit from some obscure South Sea island. Revel in the bright reds and yellows and greens and purples. Think about how lovely all those colors would look on your plate.

Next, go up and down each aisle looking at everything you see. In the frozen food section, peer into every freezer. Yes, there are a lot of meat products, but if you look closely you'll start to see vegetarian sausages, vegetarian burgers, vegetarian burritos, and whole vegetarian dinners. Take foods out and look at the labels. Imagine putting them in a cart to take home with you. Don't forget to notice all the frozen fruits and vegetables and baked goods. They can be a great help during the winter or when you don't have time to cook.

Continue down each aisle in the same manner. Look at boxes and bottles and cans. Check out the specialty food shelves: Mexican food, Chinese food, Japanese food, Indian food, dietetic and health and natural foods, gourmet foods. All of these are grist for the vegetarian mill.

If you are planning to be a lacto-ovo vegetarian, examine all the cheeses, yogurts, and other dairy products that are available to you. And whether you want to be a lacto-ovo vegetarian or a vegan, be sure to investigate the tofu and other soy products such as tempeh, miso, soy yogurt, soy cheese, soy "meats," and soy ice cream.

Finally, if your market has a deli, make a stop there. Almost any deli can make a decent vegetable sandwich, either with or without cheese. And what about salads? At the very least, most delis have potato salad, macaroni salad, pasta salad, and three-bean salad. If you're really lucky, your deli is one of those that is now carrying vegetarian burgers and a wide variety of interesting pastas, Asian noodle dishes, and even rice-and-tofu plates.

After you have finished with your regular store, try another walk through the specialty stores you discovered while doing Step Three. Look at everything they offer, too, no matter how strange. The more options you have, the more fun your new diet will be.

### That's What Friends Are For

After you have (soy) milked the grocery stores for all they are worth, you can very often find even greater inspiration among your friends and family. Thumb through the family recipe box. Ask everyone you know for their favorite vegetarian recipes (you may have to define what you mean by "vegetarian" first). At a party, you might score a great recipe for spinach lasagna from the hosts. At a potluck, you could track down a fabulous new vegan dessert someone bought at a local store. Ask your grandmother to show you how she makes that to-die-for spanikopita. Beg your next-door neighbors for their famous homemade barbecue sauce to put on your grilled tofu. The possibilities are endless.

## Other Avenues

Another great way to build up a selection of new recipes and vegetarian cooking techniques is to get a subscription to at least one of the vegetarian magazines listed in the Resources chapter. When combined with the three cookbooks I suggest you buy, you will have a selection of brand-new recipes that will keep you happy for years.

Don't give up on your old recipe sources, either. Non-vegetarian cookbooks, magazines, newspapers, and television cooking programs often have a generous number of good vegetarian recipes. You just have to look.

## Trying Them On for Size

After you have finished your exploration, go ahead and begin to systematically make the things you want to sample. If you are feeling very ambitious, this might also be a good opportunity to prepare some of the more challenging substitutes you may have skipped over when doing Step Three.

Even after you have finished the Five Steps and become a vegetarian, you will probably want to keep experimenting with new ideas. Just make sure you have something you like to eat available in case the trial is a failure!

And just as you did in the previous step, when you find something you like enough to buy or make regularly, write it in your notebook or on the pages provided for Step Four.

## The Home Stretch

This is it! The next step is the last one and after it, you will be a vegetarian! It won't take much time to do; you have already done the majority of the work. What it will take is mental preparedness and confidence, so before moving on, I urge you to search out a quiet place to contemplate this important change in your life.

**STEP FOUR:**
## My New Vegan Foods

**STEP FOUR:**
*My New Lacto-Ovo Vegetarian Foods*

# Step Five:
## Making the Change

You should be very proud of yourself. You have not only had the strength and courage to decide to become a vegetarian, but you have actually done what you had to do to make it happen. You decided that you wanted to be a vegetarian, what type of vegetarian you wanted to be, and why. You analyzed your diet, categorized it, made substitutions for parts of it, and added to it. You now have a whole new list of regularly eaten foods, perhaps much different from what you ate before. In Step Five, you will look at that new list in all its splendor!

The example for Step Five is a list of foods that consolidates the work of the other four steps. There are foods from the original lists in Steps One and Two, foods from the substitute list in Step Three, and foods from the new list in Step Four. Altogether, they make up a list of foods similar to those that might be eaten regularly by someone on either a lacto-ovo vegetarian or a vegan diet (I have omitted details such as whether the milk and cheese is from soybeans or from a cow. You should be able to fill that in yourself by now).

Please note that I have not included every food mentioned in the previous examples. In reality, most people settle down to a core list of one or two dozen items, and I have attempted to convey that in this final example. For fun, turn back to the beginning, and compare it to the example of Step One.

**STEP FIVE** *Example:*

## My List of All-Vegetarian Foods

Cereal with cow's milk or soy milk

Orange juice

Coffee

Scrambled eggs or tofu

Toast with jam

Falafel/tahini or roasted red pepper sandwich

Vegetable chow mein

Olive/mushroom pizza

Soft drinks

Apples

Carrot sticks

Jicama

Sesame-seed breadsticks

White wine

Split pea soup with French bread

Lentil dahl with potatoes

Portobello mushrooms, marinated and grilled

Mixed green salad with oil dressing

*Steamed greens: Swiss chard, collards*

*Bean and cheese tacos*

*Corn chips with salsa or bean dip*

*Mushroom-vegetable stir-fry over rice*

*Ice cream*

*Cookies*

*Fruit crumble*

## Drum Roll, Please!

Now it's time to assemble your own list and analyze it to make sure that you are fully prepared to take the final plunge into being a vegetarian. How long the final commitment takes depends on how mentally prepared you are. You have the knowledge; all you need is the desire.

Recall the date you originally set for yourself to finish the entire Five Step process. The easiest thing to do is to determine that you will become vegetarian—thereby finishing Step Five—on that date. Alternatively, you might want to pick another date, either earlier or later. When you have made your decision, write it down.

*I plan to finish Step Five by:*

_____

## Making It On Your Own

As you assemble your final list, keep in mind that it is supposed to consist of foods that you actually eat. You may very well like many other things and even eat them on occasion, but this list is for the basic everyday foods that make up the bulk of your new diet.

As in the example, some of these foods will be old standbys from the first two steps. Others will be substitutes from the third step and still others will be new foods from the fourth step. All of them will be foods you know and like and are comfortable buying, cooking, and eating.

In other words, the foods on this list will just be the foods you are currently eating, minus any non-vegetarian (or non-vegan) foods that still remain in your diet. You are merely re-analyzing your diet in exactly the same way as you did in Step One, only now you have a much larger number of vegetarian foods in your repertoire.

**STEP FIVE:**
## My List of All-Vegetarian Foods

## Checkin' It Twice

After you have filled in the worksheet, study it carefully. Does it include a wide variety of foods? Do you have favorite vegetarian breakfasts? Lunches? Dinners? Snacks? Desserts? Do you have simple things that you can whip up in a few minutes? Are there a couple of elaborate things for when you want something a little more interesting? Are there sweet things and crunchy things and light things and "meaty" things? Is this a list of foods that you can eat from and not feel deprived?

If the answer to that last question is "no," then you need to go back to Steps Three and Four. It is vital that you have a diet you can live with if you are going to succeed. Otherwise, boredom or cravings could undermine your determination. Make sure that your list contains enough foods, and a wide enough variety of foods, to satisfy you.

Of course, this doesn't mean that you will never again eat anything except what's on your list. You can continue to experiment with new vegetarian foods all the time. But you need to know that you have foods that will satisfy you now.

## The Grand Finale

To become a vegetarian, just start to eat exclusively from your list of vegetarian foods on your goal date. That's it! It really is that simple. If, from that day on, your everyday foods are from the list and you don't put any meat into your mouth again, then you are a vegetarian. Your diet will continue to evolve and change. In five years you will probably eat different foods from those you are eating now. But whatever you eat, it's your diet, and it's vegetarian.

Exactly how you make the final transition is up to you. You might have become a vegetarian before picking up this book and are simply using it to improve your diet. You might have begun eating a vegetarian diet as soon as you finished Step Two, merely using the other steps to increase your options. Or you might still be unsure about your decision and not quite ready to take that final step.

In the latter case, here are some things you can do. First, realize that your decision is not irrevocable. Some people who have been vegetarian for one or two or twelve years do return to an omnivorous diet. Usually these are people who became vegetarian for aesthetic or religious reasons, and who then had a change of beliefs. Commit yourself to eating a vegetarian diet for six months or a year after which you can decide if you want to continue.

If your motivation is still weak, re-read the reasons to become a vegetarian that were given in the introductory section. You might also spend more time perusing the materials given in the Resources. By studying up on factory farming, food distribution, nutrition, and the like, you very likely will find something that will rouse you to follow through with your commitment. There's nothing quite like having the courage of your convictions!

Of course, the aesthetic argument can be even more effective than the health and ethical ones. By deliberately developing the "eew, that's disgusting" response, you will find yourself refusing meat with a willingness you wouldn't have thought possible a short time ago!

Finally, put a copy of your list on your refrigerator where you can consult it before doing the grocery shopping. Also make a point of continuing to experiment regularly with new vegetarian foods. Every vegetarian meal you eat is a non-vegetarian meal you don't eat. Before you know it, you will have "squeezed out" your old foods in favor of the new ones. Your kitchen and your plate will be so full of vegetarian foods, you won't have the time or the appetite for anything else!

Whichever way you do it, and whenever you do it, just do it and be proud! The change you've made in your life also reflects on the rest of the world. By adopting a vegetarian diet, you are resisting personal illness, cruelty to animals, unbalanced food distribution, and damage to the planet.

# Fine-Tuning

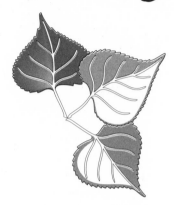

# Onward and Upward

There are many more vegetarians in our society now than there were twenty years ago. In the future, there will be still more. Even those who eat meat are eating less of it, and vegetarian foods are considered to be a growth industry. You will find that your vegetarian way of eating will get easier and easier as time goes on.

It is, however, still a meat-eating world out there, and even experienced vegetarians can get tripped up now and then. Now that you are a vegetarian, you still might need some help in order to stay that way. In the following pages, I have outlined some common problem situations and have offered some suggestions on how to deal with them.

If you run into difficulties and need more help than I have given you here, turn to the Resources chapter. Someone, somewhere, probably has the answer you need.

# Special Occasions

You are now eating a vegetarian diet on a day-to-day basis, but what about holidays and other special occasions? Many otherwise-strict vegetarians find themselves tripping up on the turkey at Thanksgiving, the gefilte fish during Passover, or the ham at Christmas. Vegans may find it difficult to avoid boiled eggs at Easter, challah on the Sabbath, milk chocolate on Halloween, and cake and ice cream at birthday parties. But with a little advanced planning there's no need to compromise yourself. You can have your holidays and your vegetarianism, too.

Here are several possible scenarios with suggestions you can adapt to your particular situation:

*You are the person to do the cooking, and you create new menus for every occasion.*

In this scenario, it's an easy matter to make the meals vegetarian. The people you invite will be prepared for new foods, so they are unlikely to raise a fuss. Finding special occasion vegetarian recipes is no harder than finding any other new recipes. Vegetarian magazines regularly feature holiday recipes, and holiday-oriented and ethnic vegetarian cookbooks are also available.

*You are not the person to do the cooking.*

There are three possible approaches here. The first is to go to the party and eat whatever vegetarian food is available. If you aren't sure what the food will be, or you know that most of it will not be acceptable to you, it might be a good idea to eat before you leave home.

The second approach is to offer to bring a dish (or two or three) with you. This works well for informal occasions and sometimes works even for formal settings, especially since special occasions are usually celebrated with close friends and family.

An extension of that idea is to become the cook. Instead of going to another person's house, offer to hold the celebration in your own home, creating your own menu. This is a lot more work, but it gives you complete control.

*You are the cook, and are expected to make the traditional dishes.*

This is the most difficult case. If you are very strong-willed and are adamant that no meat be brought into your house, you can just change the menu over other people's objections. That is almost guaranteed to generate bad feelings, however, and is not recommended for family celebrations unless your family is very open to your change of diet.

A much easier method is to turn all of the cooking over to someone else, and then act as a guest. In a very traditional family, you sometimes have more leeway as a guest than you do as the principal cook.

Another possibility is to cook all the vegetarian dishes yourself, but to ask others to bring the non-vegetarian items they want. This works well if you do not object to having meat in your home.

Finally, you can just shut your eyes and cook everything as usual and refrain from eating the meat (or lacto-ovo) items. Leftovers can then be eaten by a non-vegetarian family member or sent home with a non-vegetarian guest.

## Changing of the Guard

No matter which scenario you find yourself in, you can use the Five Step process to change a traditional holiday menu:

*Step One*
Start by writing down the foods traditionally eaten for the occasion.

*Step Two*
Split the list into two parts: Vegetarian and Non-vegetarian. Alternatively, you can use three parts: Vegan, Lacto-ovo Vegetarian, and Non-vegetarian.

*Step Three*
Search for substitutes. For example, you could make vegan pumpkin pie for Thanksgiving or buy soy hot dogs for an Independence Day barbecue.

*Step Four*
Experiment with some completely new recipes. Have a huge stuffed squash in the center of the table at Thanks-

giving or barbecue a pizza on the Fourth of July. Let your imagination fly!

*Step Five*

Write down your new list of foods for the occasion. You have created a new tradition for years to come!

# *Eating Out*

Eating everyday meals outside of the home presents another special set of challenges for vegetarians. When eating at the home of a friend, one of the ideas from the "special occasions" section should work. In the case of restaurants, airlines, and other commercial establishments, additional tricks come into play. Here are some ideas of how to approach several broad categories of institutional eateries.

## Let's Go Out to Eat

If you are like most people, you have several favorite restaurants you go to on a regular basis such as the pizzeria, the Chinese take-out, and the Mexican place down the street. During working hours, you might grab a bite for lunch at the local deli or pushcart and then entertain clients at a fancy restaurant in the evening. And some of your special occasions, such as Mother's Day or Super Bowl Sunday, might be celebrated in restaurants. Eating out is a favorite national pastime.

As a new vegetarian, you may be dismayed to find that your favorite eateries aren't up to the task of preparing good vegetarian food. Most of the fast food joints have yet to acknowledge veggie burgers, many restaurants use lard, and even the best chefs may turn out shamefully soggy and boring vegetable plates with a bit of white bread on the side.

Does being a vegetarian mean you must give up the enjoyment and practicality of restaurant dining? Not at all.

With a little time, energy, and ingenuity, eating out will soon be as simple and effortless as it was before.

A modified Five Step process can be used to develop both a list of restaurants and a list of restaurant foods that will satisfy you. I have outlined the process below.

### Step One
Make a list of your old favorite restaurants. For each of those restaurants, write down a separate list of the foods you habitually order.

### Step Two
Within each list, split the foods into two groups: Vegetarian and Non-vegetarian, or three groups: Vegan, Lacto-ovo Vegetarian, and Non-vegetarian.

### Step Three
Go to each of your restaurants and search for 1) vegetarian substitutes for your non-vegetarian favorite foods, and 2) new vegetarian foods. After perusing the menu carefully, talk to a serving person or even the cook in order to learn what the ingredients are, and to ascertain what changes can be made as well as how much advance notice they need. If you're lucky, the cook might even offer to create entirely new dishes for you or to use recipes you supply.

### Step Four
Use the Yellow Pages to look for new restaurants. Types of restaurants you might try include: Vegetarian or Health Food, Indian, Middle Eastern, Chinese, Japanese, Thai, Vietnamese, Mexican, Italian, and African. For each restaurant you try, make a list of dishes you like, similar to the lists you made in Step Three.

### Step Five
Consolidate your lists. You should end up with a new list of several restaurants that you like, as well as a list of the foods that you can order at each one.

## Cafeteria Style

If you work in a hospital, school, or business environment, you might be at the mercy of cafeteria cooks. Many food services have begun to offer salad bars as well as daily vegetarian, and even vegan, entrees, but the selection is usually poor. You may have to take action in order to get what you need.

First look to see what vegetarian food is currently available from your food service. If it is inadequate, approach the person in charge with a request for change. It is important to show respect for the food servers. They are professionals, and most of them do the best they can in a hard and thankless job.

Several vegetarian organizations have wonderful "kits" or other materials you can use when working with cafeteria people. These kits contain advice on how to best approach food service representatives. They also have information on vegetarian nutrition and ingredients as well as institutional-size recipes. With these kits, you will be able to give the meal planners and cooks exactly what they need, thereby greatly increasing your chances of success.

Of course, you can always start bringing your own food with you. There are some great vegetarian fast foods that can be popped into a microwave or heated with some boiling water. There are also many fun food containers on the market. Just plop in some leftovers, and away you go!

## Traveling Fare

All travelers have to search for food, but the vegetarian traveler sometimes needs to work a little harder. The place to start is at home before you leave.

First, let your travel agent know that you are a vegetarian or a vegan. He or she can order a special vegetarian or vegan meal for you on the airline when making your reservation. Make a note to yourself to verify your meal when confirming your flight, when checking in at the airport, and with the flight attendant before the meals are served.

Second, try to arrange to stay at places that are known to accommodate vegetarians. Many vegetarian organizations have compiled listings of vegetarian-friendly hotels, bed & breakfasts, restaurants, cruise ships, and the like. When you know your itinerary, contact the national and local vegetarian societies before you make reservations, and ask them for information about the areas you will be visiting.

Third, when you arrive at your destination look in the phone book and the tourist guides for information about restaurants. Ask the concierge for help as well. Your experience with eating out at home will come in handy when looking for eateries while traveling. Look for places similar to those you like at home. Restaurants the world over have similar menus, especially the national and international chains. The chef at the hotel may also be able to accommodate your needs if given advance notice.

Of course travelers don't have to go to restaurants all the time. You can almost always make a good and nutritious meal from the local grocery stores or open-air markets. Look for juices, breads, chips, pastries, raw or pickled vegetables, fruits, cheeses, yogurts, and canned beans. Take along a can opener, folding knife, cloth napkin, plate, cup, and set of utensils. Backpacking stores have excellent lightweight items you can buy for your kit.

Finally, many vegetarians, especially vegans, take an emergency stash of foods. Some bread and fruit can save a bad airline meal from being a total disaster (check import laws before taking produce over international borders). Dried fruit, energy bars, instant oatmeal, crackers, and peanut butter could keep you from starving in vegetarian-hostile areas. Some people even arrange to send themselves "CARE" packages when traveling in out-of-the-way places. It's just a matter of being prepared.

Last, but not least, if you don't speak the native language, I suggest you get a phrase book that has translations concerning food and eating in general and special food needs in particular. A good phrase book is essential if you are going off the beaten path, away from the tourist areas. At the very least, you will be able to say something simple like, "Fish, no. Fruit, yes," even if it does make you feel a little silly!

Berlitz Books publishes a series of phrase books which contain some translations specifically for vegetarians. Most of those books are in the classical European languages. For more exotic languages, I recommend Lonely Planet Press phrase books.

# Nutrition

As a new vegetarian, the most important thing you need to know is that humans have no nutritional need for meat, dairy products, or eggs.[1] Humans actually have no nutritional need for any particular food. What we have a need for is *nutrients*—water, carbohydrates, proteins, fats, fiber, vitamins, and minerals. Because we are omnivores those nutrients can be obtained in a variety of ways.

For millions of years, human beings have led productive lives while eating whatever foods were available to them. There were, and are, times when people have had poor diets due to a restriction in variety or quantity, but by and large our ancestors survived quite well without following any formal food groupings.

## Food Groups

In the early part of this century, food groups were devised by nutrition scientists as a simple pictorial method of encouraging people (especially poor, urban immigrants) to get the nutrients they need. The groupings were based upon the types of foods that were commonly eaten in our culture, and the main idea was that of encouraging variety, or what is often called "balance."

Since then, the United States Department of Agriculture (USDA) has promulgated many different food groupings. In 1930, there were twelve groups, followed by a reduction to seven groups in 1944. The famous (or infamous) four groups, called the Basic Four and that we are all so familiar with, came along in 1956, probably due to pressures from the burgeoning animal agriculture and processed foods industries.[2] Now, in the 1990s, we have the new Eating Right Pyramid, which is a somewhat healthier version of the four groups.

As all this shows, food groupings are not set in stone. Instead, they are a tool which can be used to obtain the variety that is the hallmark of a nutritious diet. As our knowledge of human nutritional needs grows, food groupings become more useful all the time, and several vegetarian groupings are now available. They have been summarized below to help you improve the quality of your vegetarian diet.

When a range of servings is recommended, the lower number of servings is suggested for inactive adults. Active people and pregnant or lactating women might need the higher number of servings. Also note that these recommendations are for adults. Very young children might have needs not covered by these serving suggestions. Several vegetarian nutrition books for children are listed in the Resources chapter.

Finally, remember that you don't have to eat everything every day. Most nutritionists advise that the recommendations be averaged over the course of several days or a week.[3] For example, if you have five servings of vegetables on Monday, two servings on Tuesday, and three servings on Wednesday, you will have averaged just over three servings of vegetables per day for the three days. Only when you consistently eat fewer than the recommended number of servings is there a marked need for improvement.

### The Physicians Committee's New Four Food Groups

The Physicians Committee for Responsible Medicine (PCRM) is a non-profit group of medical doctors and lay-people dedicated to improving human health through preventive medicine. Since a vegetarian diet is well suited to furthering this goal, the promotion of such a diet is a main focus of their work.

When the USDA came out with the Eating Right Pyramid which reduced the number of suggested servings for animal-based foods and vegetable fats, PCRM thought it didn't go far enough. In consequence, PCRM developed a

---

### WHAT IS A SERVING?

Your idea of a serving of a particular food may be very different from someone else's, but nutritionists have settled on some measurements that are commonly used. A standard serving, unless otherwise noted, is defined as:

*Grains:* 1 slice of bread; 1 ounce dry cereal; ½ cup cooked grain or pasta

*Vegetables:* ½ cup cooked vegetables; 1 cup raw, leafy vegetables; ½ cup raw, chopped vegetables; 4–6 ounces vegetable juice

*Fruits:* 1 medium-sized whole fruit; ½ cup cooked fruit; 4–6 ounces fruit juice

*Legumes:* ½ cup cooked legumes; 4 ounces tofu; 1 cup soy milk

*Nuts and Seeds:* 2–4 tablespoons seeds; 1 ounce nuts; or 2 tablespoons nut butter

*Dairy Products and Eggs:* 1 medium hen's egg; 1 cup cow's milk; 1 ounce cheese

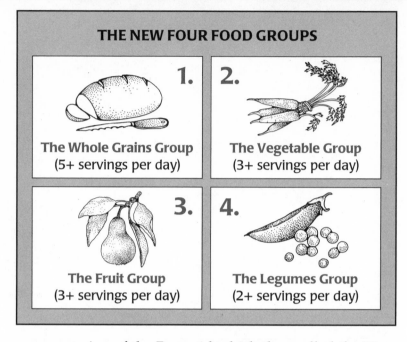

**THE NEW FOUR FOOD GROUPS**

**1.** The Whole Grains Group (5+ servings per day)

**2.** The Vegetable Group (3+ servings per day)

**3.** The Fruit Group (3+ servings per day)

**4.** The Legumes Group (2+ servings per day)

vegan version of the Pyramid which they called the New Four Food Groups. Developed in 1991, the New Four Food Groups promote better health and a lessening of the risk of heart disease, cancer, and stroke.

The President of PCRM, Neal Barnard, M.D., has written several excellent books explaining vegetarian nutrition in general and PCRM's New Four Food Groups in particular. Pamphlets and posters on vegetarian nutrition are also available from PCRM.

In addition to foods from the four groups, a reliable source of vitamin $B_{12}$ is recommended, such as fortified cereal or a supplement. Vitamin $B_{12}$ is made by microorganisms. Because much of our food has been rendered sterile due to processes such as pasteurization, $B_{12}$ may be lacking in a strict vegan diet. Supplementation is presently being recommended by many vegetarian nutritionists as a precautionary measure.

## Dr. Klaper's Vegan Six Food Groups

Dr. Michael Klaper is a medical doctor who has published several books on vegan nutrition and is also a popular guest speaker and educator. He is on the Board of Directors of the EarthSave Foundation, and much of his work is done in conjunction with that group. In his book *Vegan Nutrition: Pure and Simple,* Dr. Klaper has proposed the following grouping which he calls the Vegan Six. Please note that the serving sizes are different from those given above.

1. Whole Grains and Potatoes: 2–4 servings (4 ounces) per day
2. Legumes: 1–2 servings (3–4 ounces) per day
3. Green and Yellow Vegetables: Green: 1–2 servings (4 ounces) per day; Yellow: 1–2 servings (4 ounces) every other day
4. Nuts and Seeds: 1–3 servings (1 ounce) per day
5. Fruits: 3-6 servings per day
6. Vitamin $B_{12}$ and Mineral Foods: 1 serving of each at least three times per week. These foods include root vegetables, unwashed mushrooms, sea vegetables, and a reliable $B_{12}$ source.

## The Vegetarian Food Pyramid

A non-profit group called The Health Connection has published its own vegetarian food grouping in response to the USDA's Eating Right Pyramid. The Vegetarian Food Pyramid can be used by both vegans and lacto-ovo vegetarians since soy milk is grouped with dairy products rather than legumes, and eggs are included in the meat alternative group.

Laminated color posters of the Vegetarian Food Pyramid are available from The Health Connection, along with other materials on diet and nutrition.

1. Whole Grain Bread, Cereal, Pasta, and Rice Group: 6–11 servings per day
2. Vegetable Group: 3–5 servings per day
3. Fruit Group: 2–4 servings per day
4. Legume, Nut, Seed, and Meat Alternative (including eggs) Group: 2–3 servings per day
5. Low-fat or Non-fat Milk, Yogurt, Fresh Cheese, and Fortified Alternative (such as soy milk) Group: 2–3 servings per day

Vegetable oils and fats, sweets, and salt are to be eaten sparingly.

### The McDougall Plan

Dr. John McDougall is a medical doctor who has become an acknowledged expert on vegan nutrition. In 1986, he founded a respected health clinic at the St. Helena Hospital and Health Center in the Napa Valley of California. In addition to his clinic and his formal nutrition research, Dr. McDougall has published numerous books and cookbooks (with Mary McDougall) based upon his work.

Dr. McDougall suggests that the basic diet be composed of unlimited amounts of the following foods:

1. Whole grains and milled whole grains
2. Starchy vegetables such as potatoes, sweet potatoes, yams, and squashes
3. Yellow and green vegetables
4. Whole fruits (2–3 per day is best for most people)
5. Beans, peas, and lentils (a maximum of 1 cup a day is best)

Vegetable oils, fatty vegetables (e.g., avocado, olives), processed foods (e.g., white rice, tofu), nuts, seeds, simple sugars, and salt are discouraged, although fit and healthy individuals can usually eat small amounts of those foods without problems. A $B_{12}$ supplement is recommended.

## Alternative Eating Systems

In addition to formal food groupings, a number of different dietary philosophies have been developed. Some of these are healthy while others are more questionable. By comparing them to the above nutritional recommendations, you should be able to judge which is which. Three reasonable systems that are popular with vegetarians are described below.

## Natural Hygiene

The philosophy of natural hygiene was initially developed by several independent practitioners during the early part of the 19th century. In 1850, a group of four physicians—Sylvester Graham, William Alcott, Mary Grove, and Isaac Jennings—consolidated much of that knowledge and proceeded to teach it to others. Dr. Russell Trall formed the first national hygienic association in 1862 and wrote many important works on the subject. He was followed in this century by Dr. Herbert Shelton who shaped natural hygiene into its present form.

Natural hygiene is an overall plan for healthful living which incorporates a dietary scheme known as food combining. The idea behind food combining is that 1) certain foods do not digest properly when eaten at the same time or at the wrong time of day, and 2) certain foods are toxic to the body while others help clear toxins (waste products) from the body.

Harvey and Marilyn Diamond are modern-day proponents of the principles of natural hygiene. In their best-selling books *Fit for Life*, and *Fit for Life II: Living Health*, the Diamonds have combined the traditional rules of natural hygiene with their own experiences in a program that has enabled many people to regain their health. An explanation of the entire system is beyond the scope of this book, but a summary of the main dietary points follows:

1. Plant foods are emphasized. Because we evolved to eat plants rather than animals, natural hygienists believe our bodies cannot digest animal foods efficiently.
2. Foods should either be raw or processed as little as possible. Processing and cooking causes chemical changes in foods ("devitalizes" them) so they become disease-producing rather than health-promoting.
3. Nothing should be eaten between 8:00 pm and awakening. This spares your body the task of digesting food while you are trying to sleep as well as giving your body time to eliminate toxins.
4. Fresh fruit or fruit juices should be consumed exclusively from awakening until noon. Fruits will give you plenty of energy for the most active part of the day. At the same time, they are easy to digest and won't make you sleepy just when you need to be most awake.
5. Eat foods that contain a lot of water (i.e., fruits and vegetables). Water is desirable because it flushes toxins from the body.
6. Protein foods and starches should not be eaten during the same meal. Human stomachs do not digest proteins and starches efficiently when they are eaten together.
7. Clean (distilled) water should be drunk throughout the day except while eating or directly after a meal. Clean water flushes waste from the body, but it can impede digestion if consumed with food.

## Raw Foods

Raw foodists eat most or all of their foods in a raw, uncooked state. The theory behind the raw food philosophy is that on an evolutionary scale, cooking is a recent invention. Humans are the only animals who cook their food, and we have only been doing so for a short time in evolutionary terms. Raw foodists believe that high-heat cooking devitalizes and chemically changes foods in such a way as to cause disease.

A healthy vegetarian raw food diet is based on a wide variety of uncooked plant foods such as raw, dried, and juiced fruits and vegetables, nuts, seeds, sprouted grains, and sprouted legumes. Some people also eat raw dairy products and/or raw eggs (if you choose that option, buy certified products from a reputable supplier).

Some raw foodists, such as the followers of "instinctive nutrition therapy" (anopsotherapy), advocate eating each type of food singly and in its natural state, with no mixing, grinding, or juicing. Other raw foodists have challenged themselves to develop an elaborate cuisine which utilizes specialized heat-free or extra-low-heat cooking techniques. They are then able to make all kinds of foods such as breads, soups, salads, burgers, pizzas, dairy substitutes, cakes, puddings, and pies.

The strictest form of the natural hygiene diet is actually a type of raw food diet. It is possible, however, to eat a raw food diet and not follow the other principles of the natural hygiene school, so they are not exactly the same.

## Macrobiotics

The term "macrobiotics," which means "great-life" in Greek, has been in existence since antiquity, but the modern philosophical movement which bears the name was developed during the first part of this century by a Japanese man named Yukikazu Sakurazawa. After World War I, Sakurazawa moved to Paris, adopted the name George Ohsawa, and proceeded to devote his life to teaching others about his macrobiotic lifestyle.

Ohsawa's macrobiotics is based on Taoism, a philosophy wherein the universe is polarized into yin (passive, "feminine") and yang (active, "masculine") elements. Balance is sought between these opposing life forces. Foods are classified as either more yin or more yang depending upon an elaborate set of criteria. For example, the classification of a particular food might depend on where and how it was grown, the time of year, and whether the person eating it is male or female.

There are seven different stages of the traditional macrobiotics philosophy, with the diet for each stage becoming more and more stringent as the practitioner becomes more adept. The diets in the more advanced stages are extreme and should be avoided.[4] The basic diet is excellent, however, and many vegetarians thrive on it, with the exclusion of the occasional fish and seafood dishes.

Vegetarian macrobiotic-style meals usually begin with a soup. The main courses are based on cooked whole grains, especially rice, and regular vegetables. Sea vegetables and legumes supplement the meals while small amounts of seeds, nuts, and fruits are used as snacks or desserts. Modest portions of animal foods are sometimes included once or twice a week, which for vegetarians means occasional dairy products and eggs. The main beverages are spring water, amasake (rice milk), and various teas.

In addition, the macrobiotic philosophy calls for the use of organic and locally grown foods. Seasonings are used sparingly. Macrobiotics practitioners also have long lists of which plant foods are considered to be acceptable (e.g., broccoli, short-grain brown rice, apples) and which are to be avoided (e.g., spinach, yeasted breads, pineapple).[5] Some books on the subject have been listed in the Resources chapter.

### Consensus and Disagreement

A comparison of the above food groupings and dietary philosophies turns up some obvious similarities. The consensus appears to be that a healthful vegetarian diet is based on a wide variety of whole grains, vegetables, fruits, and legumes supplemented by small amounts of nuts and seeds, plus a B$_{12}$ source.

Everyone seems to agree that the less processed these foods are, the better, and that sweets, salt, fats, and oils are best avoided as much as possible. Whether foods are healthier when cooked or raw is a question still open for debate. A good rule-of-thumb is to eat at least one-third to one-half of the bulk (volume) of your diet as raw foods. Another good general rule is to aim for a diet composed of approximately 15 percent fat, 10 percent protein, and 75 percent carbohydrate. You can then play with these numbers until you find what feels right for you.

Disagreement also remains concerning dairy products and eggs. Most vegetarian experts agree that dairy products and eggs are not necessary, and some insist that they are downright harmful. If dairy products are eaten, low-fat or non-fat varieties are recommended. If eggs are eaten, they are probably best limited to three or four a week, including eggs in baked goods.

How you use this nutritional information is up to you. You might choose to closely follow just one of the food groupings or dietary philosophies discussed above. Alternatively, you might experiment with several different guidelines until you create a composite system all your own. As long as you don't deviate too far from the consensus position, you should be just fine.

## Getting Down to Brass Tacks

Even when following the above guidelines, there might be times when you want to emphasize a specific nutrient in your diet for some reason of your own. A brief description of the major nutrients is given below, along with examples of vegetarian sources for each one.

It is extremely difficult to overdose on any particular nutrient when it is obtained through whole plant foods. We have obviously evolved to be able to utilize such natural vitamin and mineral sources, so it is not surprising that the various nutrients in plants come "packaged" in the correct types and proportions for our bodies to use efficiently.

A corollary to this is that you should not need artificial vitamins and minerals as long as you have a varied diet of healthful foods. Vitamin and mineral pills may even upset your body's ability to utilize the nutrients naturally present in your diet by interfering with the metabolism of certain substances. Nutritional supplements are concentrated doses of specific chemicals, and mega-doses of many substances may be harmful.[6]

If your diet is not as healthful as it could be, or you are not feeling as well as you would like, I suggest you consult a vegetarian-friendly doctor or registered dietician for professional advice. If you then choose to take nutritional supplements, make sure the ingredients are from vegetarian sources and that the capsules are not made from gelatin.

You might also consider consulting a reputable herbalist. Many herbs contain concentrated amounts of certain nutrients and can be an effective source of supplementation.

## Specific Nutrients and Where to Get Them
### Protein

Protein (the eight essential amino acids) is a much overrated nutrient. Yes, we need it, but we don't need as much as was previously thought, and it's easy to get. If you eat a varied diet of whole plant foods that supplies you with adequate calories, then you are getting enough protein.[7]

Many nutrition books, including several vegetarian ones, state that vegetable proteins are inferior to animal proteins, and that plants must be properly "combined" in order to meet our nutritional needs. This is incorrect information based on out-of-date research which can safely be ignored.[8]

Even worse, too much protein may actually cause as many problems as too little! Osteoporosis, gout, and deterioration of kidney function are three serious conditions which have been linked to excessive protein consumption.[9] Concentrated protein foods should therefore be eaten in moderation. A range of 2.5 to 10 percent of calories as protein is ample for most people.[10]

Vegetarian foods that contain concentrated amounts of protein include: legumes (beans, peas, and lentils); soy products; wheat gluten (seitan); whole grains; nuts and seeds; dairy products; eggs.

## Calcium

The amount of calcium you eat is less significant than how much calcium you actually absorb or excrete. You can maximize the absorption and minimize the excretion of calcium by eating and exercising in the following way:

1. Avoid too much concentrated protein, especially animal protein.
2. Eat foods rich in vitamin C and minerals.
3. Avoid caffeine, alcohol, and tobacco.
4. Do weight-bearing exercises such as walking and weight lifting several times a week.[11,12]

Vegetarian foods that contain large amounts of calcium include: legumes; calcium-precipitated tofu; calcium-fortified orange juice; dark, leafy greens such as kale and broccoli; sesame seeds and tahini; dried figs; dairy products. Ironically, and contrary to popular opinion, dairy products may actually contribute to calcium loss even though cow's milk contains so much calcium. This net calcium loss is thought to occur because the body strives to balance the acidity of the animal proteins with the alkalinity of the calcium.[13,14]

## Iron

Too little iron can cause anemia. If your doctor has diagnosed dietary-deficiency anemia, increase your consumption of iron-rich foods and cook in cast-iron pans. You also might try eliminating dairy products. In addition to having almost no iron, dairy products may also cause iron to be depleted from the body through an allergic response which causes intestinal bleeding.[15]

Alternatively, an excessive amount of iron in the body has recently been implicated in heart disease.[16] If your doctor has identified this as a problem for you, try reducing the amount of iron-rich foods in your diet and avoid cooking in cast-iron pans until the problem has abated.

Vegetarian foods that are rich in iron include: legumes; nuts and seeds; whole grains; blackstrap molasses; dark, leafy greens.

### Vitamin A

Our bodies turn beta-carotene into vitamin A, which helps fight infection and improves tissue and skin texture. Supplemental vitamin A is stored in the body and can become toxic in large amounts, so it is generally best to avoid vitamin A supplements.[17]

Rich sources of beta-carotene include: sweet potatoes; carrots; winter squashes; dark, leafy greens; apricots.

### Vitamins $B_1$, $B_2$, $B_3$, $B_6$

The B vitamins are essential for proper metabolic functioning. These vitamins are not stored in the body, so it is important to eat foods rich in the B vitamins every day.

Good sources of the full spectrum of B vitamins (except $B_{12}$) include: whole grains; most fruits and vegetables; yeast.

### Vitamin $B_{12}$

Vitamin $B_{12}$ is made by microorganisms such as bacteria. $B_{12}$ is essential for the health of the central nervous system. Animals, as once our own ancestors did, obtain $B_{12}$ through the dirt and grime on food they consume in the great outdoors. Our highly sanitized society has made it a bit harder for us to get this vitamin if we choose not to eat any animal products.

Fortunately, the amount of $B_{12}$ needed is minuscule, and our bodies store it for a long time. We may even have bacteria in our mouths and intestines that manufacture it, but the research is still uncertain.

To be on the safe side, strict vegans and pregnant or lactating vegetarians are being advised to regularly include a reliable source of vitamin $B_{12}$ in their diets.[18] Please note, however, that $B_{12}$ supplements can contain analogs which are not the nutrient we need, and which may actually cause the very $B_{12}$ deficiency they are designed to avert![19] If you take $B_{12}$ supplements, make sure you get them from a reputable supplier, and if you have any doubts, ask your physician to test your $B_{12}$ level.

Good vegetarian sources of vitamin $B_{12}$ include: $B_{12}$-fortified nutritional yeast; $B_{12}$-fortified cereals; $B_{12}$ vitamin tablets; eggs. Traditionally fermented miso, tempeh, and soy sauce, as they are produced in the U.S. today, are not considered to be reliable $B_{12}$ sources.[20]

### Vitamin C

Vitamin C is used by the body to build various body structures. Like the B vitamins, it is not stored in the body, so some should be eaten every day. This vitamin can be destroyed by cooking, so it is best to eat vitamin C foods in raw, or nearly raw, form.

Good vitamin C sources include: citrus fruits; dark leafy greens; tomatoes.

### Vitamin D

This is the vitamin that is not a vitamin. We make it in our own bodies when we expose our skin to the sun. If you never go outside, have dark skin, or live near the poles, you might consider a supplement. Supplemental vitamin D can be toxic in large doses, however, so it is best to instead expose your face and arms to the sun for an average of fifteen to thirty minutes a day.[21] To avoid overexposure to potentially harmful rays, you can schedule your "sun-time" for the morning or late afternoon hours.

Precursors of vitamin D are supplied by: yeast; plants.

### Vitamin E

Vitamin E is an important anti-oxidant and is also used by the body in the manufacture of muscle tissue.

Good sources of vitamin E include: whole grains; dark, leafy greens.

### Minerals

The human body uses a multitude of minerals—boron, phosphorus, magnesium, potassium, sodium, zinc, etc. A varied diet of whole plant foods, such as that recommended above, contains plentiful amounts of them all.[22]

Rich sources of minerals include: legumes; whole grains; fruits; dark, leafy greens; sea vegetables.

## Becoming a Vibrant Vegetarian

If you want to bring your vegetarian diet into line with the recommendations, you can once again use the Five Step process to help you do so. Just as you replaced your old non-vegetarian foods with vegetarian foods, so now you will gradually drop less healthful vegetarian foods in favor of more healthful ones.

You might find that it takes some time to wean yourself from your favorite, but not-so-healthful, vegetarian foods. Changing from beef hot dogs to soy hot dogs was probably not too difficult. But if you want to eat the healthiest possible vegetarian diet, you will need to eliminate the soy hot dogs from your everyday diet as well.

Remember the previous example of changing from whole-fat milk to low-fat milk? This is the same process. You will educate your palate to prefer brown rice to white rice and whole fruits to sweetened fruit drinks. You will also teach yourself to like more vegetables, plain water, and other healthful foods. Your body will undoubtedly assist you by feeling good when you eat well, and feeling bad when you eat badly. In response, you will, with time, find yourself craving the healthful foods and rejecting the unhealthful ones.

Don't become discouraged if this adjustment takes a while. Just keep in mind that every little bit helps. As Dr. John McDougall is fond of saying, "the more you do, the more you gain."

### Step One

Start with the list of foods you eat now. This will probably be the list from the end of the original Five Step process that led to your becoming a vegetarian.

### Step Two

Using the discussion of food groupings above, break your list into two parts: Healthful Vegetarian Foods and Unhealthful Vegetarian Foods. Foods which accord with the recommendations will go into the first list while the others go into the second list.

Let's look at an example. Oatmeal is a healthful whole grain cereal. If you love oatmeal, you can cheerfully place it in your list of healthful vegetarian foods. Soy sausages, on the other hand, are a highly refined and processed food. They are healthier than pork sausages because they do not contain cholesterol and often have less fat, but they still cannot be considered a truly healthful food. Soy sausages would therefore go into the list of unhealthful vegetarian foods.

### Step Three

Search for healthful substitutes for your unhealthful foods. There are foods for which there are no truly healthful substitutes, such as the soy sausages mentioned above. There are others for which the substitute bears little or no resemblance to the original. For instance, you could start putting fruit-spread on your toast instead of butter or you could even eat your toast plain.

In addition, some substitutes are simple, such as replacing white rice with brown rice. Others take more care. You might, for example, want to learn how to make your pancakes with whole-wheat flour, soy milk, and egg-replacer instead of white flour, cow's milk, and eggs. How elaborate your substitutions are is up to you.

### Step Four

Explore all new healthful foods. You have probably already done a large amount of exploration, so this shouldn't be really difficult. You might want to buy a few more cookbooks which specialize in cuisines such as raw foods or macrobiotics or which emphasize a specific technique such as juicing or a specific type of food such as vegetables or beans.

As you try new recipes, keep in mind that you need to be open to reeducating your palate to accept less fat, less sugar, and less salt. As before, try to find at least ten new foods and recipes which you like enough to regularly buy and make.

### Step Five

Compile your new list of healthful vegetarian foods. *Voilà!* You now have a truly nutritious vegetarian diet.

## Healthy Is as Healthy Does

A well-balanced diet is the keystone to good health, but you can do many other things to strengthen the positive effects of your new diet. The following list of common sense routines is adapted from the material in the Diamonds' book, *Fit for Life II: Living Health.*

1) Eat your meals at a regular time and place.
2) Get enough, but not too much, relaxation and sleep.
3) Exercise moderately with a combination of aerobics, strength training, and stretching.
4) Cultivate strong relationships with your friends and family.
5) Learn to meditate.

## *(Not) For Vegans Only*

If you have changed your diet for ethical reasons, you may also want to alter some other, non-dietary, consumption habits. Many people are clearing their closets of leather and fur or are cleaning their homes and bodies with products that were not tested on animals. Now that your diet is cruelty-free, what could be easier than changing these other habits as well?

Many animal rights and vegan organizations have compiled lists of cruelty-free products. Call them, and have them send you information on whatever items you want to change. Then set aside a day to go through your closets or cupboards with list in hand.

To help you change these other consumption habits, I have put together a generalized version of the original Five Step process which you used to change your diet. The example below illustrates how you can use this generalized procedure to change your wardrobe. You can then adapt this idea to change whatever set of items you wish.

*Step One:* Pile all the items in question on a table or bed.

*Step Two:* Separate the items according to the obvious criteria. Your wardrobe, for example, could be separated into clothes made from animals and clothes made from plants or synthetics.

*Step Three:* Go shopping! Look for substitutes for items you want to get rid of. If a belt is made of leather you might search for a belt made of canvas. A fashionable coat filled with synthetic down could take the place of your old fur.

*Step Four:* Go shopping again! Look for completely new items. For example, many towns now have stores that exclusively sell cruelty-free products and all-cotton or all-synthetic clothing.

*Step Five:* Put your new purchases away along with any old, unoffending items. In order to avoid waste, you might decide to "use up" the offending items rather than throw them away. The choice is yours, but chances are you will feel better once you have removed all the animal-origin items from your home and wardrobe.

# Other Considerations

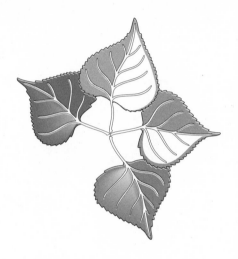

# Social Interactions

When you first told your friends and family that you were going to become a vegetarian, you probably experienced a whole range of reactions. Some people probably reacted with joy, some with interest, some with indifference—and some with hostility.

Food is more than mere nourishment for people. Meals are often a symbol of togetherness, friendship, love, and cultural belonging. A drastic change in diet can therefore be traumatic for those who are close to you. Vegetarianism challenges a whole set of assumptions about life that many in our society hold dear.

An example might serve to make this more clear. I once met a vegetarian whose father is a butcher. Such a situation will obviously be tense, at best. At worst, it could lead to a complete breakdown in communication that is agonizing for everyone involved.

Hostile reactions can cause many problems for the fledgling vegetarian. You are making what you feel is a positive step in your life, and upon sharing it with your loved ones, you are perhaps attacked and even vilified. That is the last thing anyone needs when making a big change. Learning to deal with other people in a calm, soothing, but forthright manner is therefore imperative.

The first, and most important, lesson you must learn is DO NOT PROSELYTIZE! No matter how much you love your new diet, no matter how much healthier you are, and no matter how strongly you feel about the ethical issues involved, you must remember that not everybody is open to hearing about it. This does not mean you can't be an agent of change if you so desire; it merely means that you must cultivate a winning strategy.

Start by fostering relationships with those people who are happy about your dietary change. This will give you the psychological support base from which you can reach out to those who aren't so happy with you. If there isn't a single person you can turn to among your usual social circle, I strongly suggest you join a vegetarian society and subscribe to a vegetarian magazine. Forming a network of supportive people who share your beliefs is crucial!

Once you are feeling secure, you can start to reach out to those people who are truly interested. It might take some trial and error to weed out the "fakes." Some people may exercise their animosity by pretending an interest they do not feel. Their questions are designed to trip you up rather than to enlighten anyone. Don't allow them to do that. Just say, "If you really are interested, I'd be happy to discuss it with you. But if you aren't, I would rather talk about something else."

Truly curious people are something else again. Answer their questions the best you can. If they express interest, you can lend them books and magazines or give them lists of references. But be careful not to overdo. If they show signs of resistance or restlessness, back off. It is far more important to cultivate the friendship than it is to force an instant conversion. Even if they never become vegetarian, they can still offer you valuable support.

One caveat: if for some reason you don't want to answer anyone's questions, then don't. Just because you are a vegetarian doesn't mean you have to be an activist, and even if you are an activist, it doesn't mean you have to be "on call" to everyone all the time. Practice saying, "I would love to talk to you about it sometime, but not right now," or "I prefer not to discuss my diet with anyone. If you want to learn more, I suggest you contact our local vegetarian society."

Argumentative people are best avoided if at all possible. If the person is a casual acquaintance, you can usually sidestep the issue with a simple, "I don't wish to discuss it." If he or she persists, firmly change the subject. If that doesn't work, then remove yourself from his presence, perhaps with the aid of a more sympathetic friend.

If the hostile person is a co-worker or employer, and he continues to harass you, the situation is probably best dealt with through your workplace's conflict-resolution procedures.

At home, you must go more gently. Friends and family members usually eat together often, which makes it difficult to avoid problems. The situation will be exacerbated if you are the primary food preparer. Since you are the one who has changed, you would do well to lead the way in resolving any conflict.

Start by realizing the importance of not discussing the issue of vegetarianism over the dinner table. It is also best to approach people singly because a group might gang up on you. Choose a neutral place and time for the discussion after you have both eaten and with no food present.

Make it clear that you will not tolerate antagonistic behavior during your discussion. If tempers rise despite your best efforts, go into another room until things have cooled down. In a very bad situation, you might even consider going to a third party such as a mutual friend or a professional counselor.

Reassure the person that your change of diet is not a judgement upon him. Emphasize that you care for him just as much as before. Tell him that you are doing this for yourself, and that it makes you feel good.

Then ask him why he is so unhappy with the change. Does he think you're criticizing his beliefs or behavior or line of work? If you are the primary food preparer, is he afraid that you won't cook the foods he likes anymore? Is he afraid that it might presage other, even more radical, changes? Is he afraid of what other people will think? Does he think you will convert (or subvert) the children? Does he think your shared social life will be adversely affected? Is he afraid you will leave? Is he afraid that you will become weak or sick?

Your goal is not to convert this person, but to reach a place where you can live together peaceably. Try to hammer out an arrangement you both can abide by. This will probably entail an agreement not to discuss food as well as possible compromises concerning food preparation and child rearing.

Whether at work or at home, it's possible that in a few extreme cases, no agreement will be reached. The strongest relationship can be irrevocably damaged when one party has a radical change in beliefs or habits which the other person cannot accept. Occasionally, vegetarians have found that they either have to give up and become omnivorous again or they have to allow the friendship, the job, or even the marriage to dissolve.

I sincerely hope your vegetarianism is a source of happiness for you and all who care for you. Fortunately, vegetarianism is rapidly gaining greater acceptance in our society, which can only help smooth the way. If you have a difficult situation, however, and need more help than I offer here, I urge you to read *The New Vegetarians* by Paul Amato and Sonia Partridge. A sociological study of vegetarianism and its effects on relationships and lives, Amato and Partridge's book will let you know you are not alone.

## Questions and Answers

As a vegetarian, you will undoubtedly be asked a number of common questions, most of them concerning ethics and health. If the person who asks the question seems to be truly interested, and/or you are in the mood to talk, then you might find this section useful.

*Why did you become a vegetarian?*

You answered this question at the beginning of this book. Summarizing your reasons so they can be presented in a simple sentence or two without stuttering can be helpful. For example, you might say something like, "I became a vegetarian for health reasons. Since then, I've learned about the impact my diet has on the environment and other people, which has helped me stick with it."

If the questioner wants to know more, you must decide if you want to answer in more detail. Just make sure you have your facts correct before you plunge in!

*Do you really think eating meat is wrong?*

How you answer this depends on why you became a vegetarian. If, for example, you think eating meat is perfectly all right, but you don't eat it because it makes you feel sick, then say so. Most people find that a perfectly acceptable reason because it doesn't challenge their own habits or beliefs.

If, on the other hand, you believe that animals have rights that preclude raising and killing them to eat, you would be wise to judge your questioner before answering. Usually it is safe to quietly say, "I do not wish to hurt or kill animals for my own sustenance or pleasure." Where the conversation goes after that depends on your questioner and how much of an activist you wish to be.

*Where do you get your (protein, iron, calcium)?*

The best answer is a short list of foods that are good sources of the specific nutrient mentioned. Turn to the section on nutrition for such a list. For more detail, a good vegetarian nutrition book is invaluable.

If the questioner is unconvinced, firmly state as many times as necessary, "There is no nutritional need for animal products. Every nutrient needed by humans is available from plant foods." If she persists, offer to lend her a book on the subject and close the conversation.

*Aren't you afraid your children will be malnourished?*

All parents, whether omnivorous or vegetarian, probably have some concern about their children's health and nutrition. However, vegetarianism, per se, is not a problem for anyone, no matter what their age. Several books on vegetarian nutrition for children are listed in the Resources chapter. The basics are as follows:

Babies are usually best off with breast milk or a soy-based formula. Well-mashed plant foods such as cooked cereal, bananas, and sweet potatoes are introduced in the usual manner when weaning begins at around six months. More solid foods are gradually added to the diet during the next year until the child is completely weaned. The child will then be perfectly well nourished on the same well-balanced vegetarian diet his parents eat, with the addition, during his early growing years, of a judicious amount of higher fat, less fibrous foods such as peanut butter, avocado, fruit juice, white bread, and white rice.

To illustrate: Does the omnivorous child who lives on sugared cereals and soft drinks and fast-food hamburgers have a healthier diet than the vegetarian child who eats oatmeal and orange juice and tofu burgers? Of course not. A junk-food diet is unhealthy. A varied, whole-foods, plant-based diet is healthy. Whether the diet is omnivorous or vegetarian is beside the point.

Persistent questioners again need to be firmly told that there is no nutritional need for animal products at any time past weaning. If that doesn't convince them, you can either offer more details, lend them a book on vegetarian nutrition for children, or refuse to discuss it further.

*How come you have a cold (cancer, heart disease) if you're a vegetarian?*

A major problem with the "vegetarianism is healthy" argument is that any vegetarian who suffers from an illness is likely to be challenged. The best defense is to point out that abstention from animal foods does not confer immunity from viruses, bacteria, environmental contaminants, genetic disorders, or psychological problems. Nor does it necessarily cure previously existing conditions. Finally, a vegetarian who is more concerned with ethics than health might not be eating a particularly healthy vegetarian diet.

You might mention that several studies have found that vegetarians tend to have somewhat stronger immune systems than omnivores, and so might be less prone to develop certain infectious illnesses.[1] Long-term vegetarians also are less prone to the "diseases of excess." But you should emphasize that the healthiest individual can become ill if the body's defenses are overcome.

*Don't you feed your cat (ferret, snake) meat?*

Most domesticated animals either already eat a diet of plants (e.g., rabbits, horses) or are omnivores (e.g., dogs, rats) who can easily be fed a plant-based diet. If you have a carnivorous animal in your household, however, you will be called on it.

The only possible answer is, "Yes. My pet is a carnivore. My responsibility to him requires that I feed him meat." How this is interpreted hinges on whether or not you have stated that you think eating meat is wrong. If you are a vegetarian for personal health reasons, you won't be accused of hypocrisy. If, however, you are an animal activist, you might find it useful to liberally salt your remarks with the phrase "for humans" as in, "I think it is wrong for humans to eat meat." You might also consider avoiding carnivorous companion animals in the future! (Vic Sussman, in his book *The Vegetarian Alternative*, points out that although other animals may be herbivores or frugivores, they cannot properly be called "vegetarians" because vegetarianism implies a choice rather than a biological imperative.)

It should be noted that it is theoretically possible to feed a cat a vegetarian diet through careful meal preparation and supplementation.[2] If you want to try this with your cat, I urge you to research the subject thoroughly first.

### You wear leather shoes, don't you?

Once again, this question isn't a problem for the health vegetarian who doesn't think meat eating is wrong, but if you are an ethical vegetarian, you will probably want to prepare an answer.

While you are new to vegetarianism, you might point out that you are in transition and haven't gotten around to worrying about clothing yet. After you have been a vegetarian for awhile, you can then develop your position in more detail.

Many environmentalist vegetarians, for example, wear leather because they consider it to be kinder to the environment than synthetics. This actually is not true, but most people will consider it to be a legitimate reason, nonetheless.*

---

* The environmental problems associated with raising animals for meat hold for leather, too. In the argument against using or wearing petroleum-based synthetics, it should be recalled that modern animal agriculture uses so much petroleum that meat and leather could almost be considered to be petroleum "products." In addition, the chemicals used in tanning are among the worst pollutants of our water. Although raw skin is biodegradable, leather is no longer just skin and can take decades, if not centuries, to break down. Leather is to skin as pressure-treated lumber is to a tree!

If you are an animal activist, you could point out that all your new shoes are non-leather, but you kept the old ones so as not to be wasteful. Or maybe your synthetic shoes just fooled the questioner, and you can cheerfully point out that you aren't actually wearing any leather at all!

## *Personal Adjustments*

You now have some ideas for helping others adjust to your new diet. But what about you? No matter how happy you are and how good you feel about this change in your life, there will still undoubtedly be moments when you aren't so sure. Learning to work your way through such times is an important part of the vegetarian journey.

### The Big Mac Attack

Cravings have been the downfall of a multitude of vegetarians. Benjamin Franklin, for instance, gave in to a pan of frying fish after several years as a vegetarian. What do you do when those cravings strike? The answer depends on you.

If you are determined to strictly adhere to your vegetarian diet, two paths are open to you when temptation occurs. First, there is good old-fashioned will power. How well this works for you will largely depend on your reasons for being a vegetarian. If you have strong ethical beliefs, you will probably only be momentarily tempted. After an initial moment of desire, you will remember your reasons, and the moment will pass. The longer you are a vegetarian, the easier this will become, and the moments of temptation will very likely become fewer with time.

The second method relies on your work during Steps Three and Four of the Five Step process. Instead of resisting temptation altogether, you can redirect it. Often a craving is really a desire for a particular nutrient or for emotional sustenance.[3,4] By identifying why you crave a particular non-vegetarian food, you can then search for a vegetarian food that will do the same thing. A craving for meat might just be your body's desire for iron, and some blackstrap molasses or broccoli could do the trick. A desire for ice cream might signal a need for comforting, and so a bowl of Tofutti, or a hug, could be just what you require.

## Falling off the Wagon

That brings us to the other possible response, which is giving in. If you are casual about your vegetarianism, this might not be a problem for you. You might be perfectly happy eating a vegetarian diet for ten years straight, having two slices of turkey for Thanksgiving in the eleventh year, and then going back to your vegetarian diet for another ten years with no feelings of guilt whatsoever.

Or you could decide, although I hope you don't, that after several months or years of being vegetarian your reasons are not what they were, and that after eating meat (or milk or eggs) again you don't wish to continue being a vegetarian (or a vegan).

The problems start if you become so upset over your "failure" that you feel guilty for days, or even weeks or years. This reaction is common in people who have strong ethical beliefs about vegetarianism, especially religious or animal rights beliefs.

Remember when I advised you not to proselytize about your new diet? I used the word "proselytize" for a reason. Ethical vegetarianism is more akin to a religion than a food choice. For some people, it is a part of their religion. In this case, giving in to a craving for meat (or milk or eggs) is very much like a "sin," including the guilt which accompanies such "sinfulness." If you experience such guilt after giving in to a craving, it is imperative that you deal with it in a rational manner.

Think of it as a learning experience. It isn't that your feelings of guilt are wrong. It is perfectly fine, even healthy, to feel shame when doing something you consider immoral. What is dangerous is to wallow in your feelings of guilt.

The best course is to openly acknowledge to yourself, and perhaps to others who witnessed the lapse, that you did something that you are ashamed of and to vow to do better in the future. Analyze what occurred, and figure out how you could act differently in similar circumstances. Then let it go and move on. In that way, you will strengthen your commitment to your beliefs.

### Eating Disorders

A change of diet is a big change for anybody, but for some people it is a bigger change than it is for others. If you suffer from an eating disorder, you may find that your new diet helps you overcome your problem. On the other hand, you may find that your new diet actually exacerbates your symptoms. If that is the case, it behooves you to work to overcome your psychological and/or physical problems with food.

If your eating disorder is severe, if you are suffering from malnutrition, or if your disorder is a symptom of psychological problems, I strongly suggest you contact a vegetarian-friendly physician and/or mental health professional who specializes in eating disorders. Trying to overcome your problem on your own may be very difficult or even dangerous.

I, myself, am the victim of an eating disorder. It is my firm opinion that the problems with food experienced by many people, and especially women, in this country are the result of a combination of inappropriate foods and impossible societal standards. On the one hand, we are told to eat highly processed, nutrient poor, fatty foods such as meat, dairy products, eggs, sugar, and white flour. On the other hand, we are encouraged to keep our weight below what is normal and healthy for our bodies.

The good news is that you can learn to relate to food in a healthful way. As you begin to eat a nutritious vegetarian diet, your body, and your mind, will gradually regain its chemical balance. At the same time, psychological work can help you improve your diet still further. This positive feedback system is the road to regaining your health.

During this process, the most important thing you can do for yourself is to understand that YOU ARE NOT TO BLAME FOR YOUR EATING DISORDER. Blame the government and dieticians for pushing the Four Food Groups. Blame the food processors for removing all the nutrients from the foods they make. Blame the advertisers for all those air-brushed pictures of undernourished waifs. But don't blame yourself.

## Overeating and Compulsive Eating

If you overeat, you have already taken a very important step to overcoming your problem by becoming a vegetarian. The calorie count of the high-fat, low-fiber, traditional American diet can be very high. A nutritious vegetarian diet, on the other hand, can end overeating simply by filling your stomach with bulky, fibrous foods. You get full sooner, and stay full longer.

Overeating might also be a signal that you are malnourished or your diet is unbalanced. If you choose nutrient-poor foods, your body could be starved for specific nutrients, and the system which regulates your hunger drive might not be turning off. You then continue to experience cravings even though your stomach is bursting with food. You may very well find yourself eating much less as you increase the "nutrient density" of your diet through eating lots of whole grains, fruits, and vegetables.[5]

Compulsive eating occurs when you overeat for psychological reasons. Compulsive eaters abuse food in much the same way as an alcoholic abuses liquor. Unfortunately, the reasons for your abuse of food will probably remain even after you become a vegetarian. You might even find that a vegetarian diet triggers overeating. If you feel that you are being deprived of favorite foods, you might overeat other foods to compensate.

If this is the case, you must not expect perfection from yourself. Don't let your vegetarianism become another diet, where you beat yourself up anytime you eat the "wrong" food. Instead, listen to your body. Feed it healthy foods when you can, unhealthy foods when you must, and pay attention to how each makes you feel. With time, your body will learn which foods make it feel good, and you will begin to crave them.

At the same time, you need to work on the psychological reasons for your overeating behavior. You may even need to go back to a modified omnivorous (or lacto-ovo) diet for awhile until you have worked through your problems. I highly recommend the books *Diets Still Don't Work* by Bob Schwartz and *Overcoming Overeating* by Jane Hirschmann and Carol Munter. I also urge you to seek professional counseling.

## Bulimia

Bulimia usually starts out of fear of gaining weight. It is almost impossible not to gain weight when overeating animal products. It is equally impossible to lose weight on such a diet without reducing your caloric intake. But your body has been designed by millions of years of evolution to survive, so the hunger urge soon overwhelms your "will power." What follows is a horrid cycle of starvation, binging, and purging.

By satisfying your very real hunger drive with high-fiber, low-fat, nutrient-dense foods, you can break the cycle and regain your health. If you have suffered from bulimia for some time, however, you may need more help. The physical abuse can easily turn into emotional abuse as you blame yourself and punish your body for your perceived lack of discipline. Continual binging and purging signals a need for counseling if you are to avoid malnutrition and permanent damage to your digestive system. You also might consider using the books mentioned above.

## Anorexia

If you are anorectic, you have taken the fear of weight gain to an even greater extreme. You have perfected the art of starvation while having the strength of will to resist your body's strong urge to eat. This control is a very important part of the anorectic disorder and often becomes the reason for its persistence.[6] Loss of control is more frightening to the anorectic than loss of health or even life. Anorexia is therefore a dangerous disorder which needs to be treated professionally.

Anorectics have been known to use a vegetarian diet as a method of starvation. Just as many vegetarian foods can aid in weight loss for the average person, so can they be used by anorectics to starve themselves further. This is why many health professionals who work with anorectics view a vegetarian diet with alarm. If you are vegetarian for ethical reasons, be sure to let your doctor know. Your therapy might then include higher calorie vegetarian foods such as tofu, avocado, and peanut butter rather than meat and other animal products.

# The Thousandth Mile

You have journeyed far since you first picked up this book. Many people would like to become vegetarian, but you have actually had the determination to turn your dream into reality. A person who does that is always very special, and you have every right to be proud.

And just as a stone thrown into a pond produces ever-expanding ripples, so will you now gently influence the people around you, merely through living your vegetarian life. This is a gift you give not only to yourself, but to your friends and family, and everyone else with whom you share the Earth. Even better, it is a gift you will continue to give, every day of your life, so long as you continue along this vegetarian path.

I am honored to have assisted you on your journey. You began by taking one single step. Now that you have reached the end of the thousandth mile, I extend my most heartfelt congratulations and wish you well!

# Resources

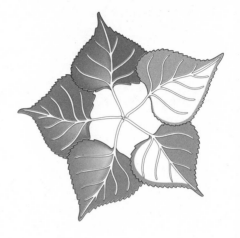

# Recommended Reading

The following lists provide a good overview of the subject of vegetarianism, but are by no means comprehensive. There are now hundreds, if not thousands, of books and other resource materials available. I have for the most part chosen books that are considered classics. Some of the lesser known titles are books which I personally like. Use these lists as a starting point in your search for further understanding and appreciation of your new diet.

If you have difficulty finding the book you want through your local bookseller, you can often mail-order through a vegetarian or animal rights group. I highly recommend the Mail Order Catalog, which has an extensive book list (see Mail Order Food Sources).

## All-Stars

If you have limited time and/or money, I highly recommend this short list of books and magazines for a good basic understanding of the subject of vegetarianism. You will find more detailed information on these materials in the lists on the following pages, where they are marked with a ☆.

☆ *The McDougall Plan* (health and nutrition)
☆ *Diet for a New America* (health and ethics)
☆ *Animal Factories* (economics and ethics)

☆ *The New Vegetarians* (sociology/psychology)
☆ *The New Laurel's Kitchen* (lacto-ovo cookbook)
☆ *Simply Vegan* (vegan cookbook)
☆ *Field of Greens* (gourmet cookbook)
☆ *Vegetarian Times* (magazine)

## Cookbooks
### Lacto-Ovo Vegetarian Cookbooks
Callan, Ginny. *Horn of the Moon Cookbook*. Harper & Row, 1987.

Hoshijo, Kathy. *Kathy Cooks: Vegetarian, Low Cholesterol*. Simon & Schuster, 1989.

Katzen, Mollie. *The Moosewood Cookbook*. Ten Speed Press, 1992.

Katzen, Mollie. *Still Life With Menu*. Ten Speed Press, 1988.

Madison, Deborah. *The Savory Way*. Bantam, 1990.

Madison, Deborah and Edward Espe Brown. *The Greens Cookbook*. Bantam Books, 1987.

☆ Robertson, Laurel and Carol Flinders and Brian Ruppenthal. *The New Laurel's Kitchen*. Ten Speed Press, 1986.

☆ Sommerville, Annie. *Field of Greens*. Bantam Books, 1993.

### Vegan Cookbooks
Hagler, Louise and Dorothy R. Bates, eds. *The New Farm Vegetarian Cookbook*. The Book Publishing Co., 1988.

Klaper, Michael, M.D., *The Cookbook for People Who Love Animals*. Gentle World, 1990.

McDougall, John, M.D. and Mary McDougall. *The New McDougall Cookbook*. NAL-Dutton, 1993.

Newkirk, Ingrid and the staff of People for the Ethical Treatment of Animals. *The Compassionate Cook: Or Please Don't Eat the Animals!* Warner Books, 1993.

Nishimoto, Miyoko. *The Now and Zen Epicure*. The Book Publishing Co., 1991.

Picarski, Brother Ron. *Friendly Foods*. Ten Speed Press, 1991.

☆ Wasserman, Debra and Reed Mangels. *Simply Vegan*. The Vegetarian Resource Group, 1991.

### Macrobiotic Cookbooks

Brown, Judy and Dorothy R. Bates. *Judy Brown's Guide to Natural Foods Cooking*. The Book Publishing Co., 1989.

McCarty, Meredith. *FRESH from a Vegetarian Kitchen*. Turning Point Publications, 1989.

Michell, Keith. *Practically Macrobiotic*. Healing Arts Press, 1988.

### Raw Foods Cookbooks

Levin, James, M.D. and Natalie Cederquist, *Vibrant Living*. GLO, Inc., 1993.

Hutchings, Imar, ed. *The Joy of Not Cooking: Vegetarian Cuisine Cooked Only by the Sun*. Delights of the Garden Press, 1994.

Kendall, Frances. *Sweet Temptations Natural Dessert Book*. Avery Publishing Group, 1988.

Meyerowitz, Steve. *Recipes from the Sproutman*. The Sprout House (PO Box 1100, Great Barrington, MA 01230, 800-777-6881), 1992.

### Ethnic Cookbooks

Devi, Yamuna. *Lord Krishna's Cuisine: The Art of Indian Vegetarian Cooking*. Bala Books, 1987.

Jaffrey, Madhur. *Madhur Jaffrey's World-of-the-East Vegetarian Cooking*. Alfred A. Knopf, 1986.

The Moosewood Collective. *Sundays at Moosewood Restaurant: Ethnic and Regional Recipes from the Cooks at the Legendary Restaurant*. Simon & Schuster, 1990.

Wasserman, Debra. *The Lowfat Jewish Vegetarian Cookbook*. Vegetarian Resource Group, 1993.

Wells, Troth. *The World in Your Kitchen*. The Crossing Press, 1993.

### Specialty Cookbooks

Cole, Candia Lea. *Not Milk . . . Nut Milks!* Woodbridge Press, 1990.

Davis, Karen. *Instead of Chicken, Instead of Turkey*. The Book Publishing Co., 1993.

Friedman, Rose. *Allergy Free Vegetarian Cookbook*. Thorson's, 1993.
McCune, Kelly. *Vegetables on the Grill*. Harper Perennial, 1992.
McNair, James. *James McNair's Vegetarian Pizza*. Chronicle Books, 1993.
Shurtleff, William and Akiko Aoyagi. *The Book of Tofu*. Ballantine Books, 1987.
Stepaniak, Joanne. *The UnCheese Cookbook*. The Book Publishing Co., 1994.

### Special Occasions Cookbooks
Atlas, Nava. *Vegetarian Celebrations*. Little, Brown, & Co., 1990.
Elliot, Rose. *Rose Elliot's Vegetarian Christmas: Festive Feasts for All the Family*. Harper Collins, 1995.

### Baking Books
Brown, Edward Espe. *The Tassajara Bread Book*. Shambala, 1986.
The Cooperative Whole Grain Education Association. *Uprisings: The Whole Grain Baker's Book*. The Book Publishing Co., 1990.
Robertson, Laurel with Carol Flinders and Bronwen Godfrey. *The Laurel's Kitchen Bread Book: A Guide to Whole-Grain Baking*. Random House, 1984.

## Nutrition
### General
Barnard, Neal, M.D. *Food for Life: How the New Four Food Groups Can Save Your Life*. Crown Publishers, 1994.
_____. *The Power of Your Plate*. The Book Publishing Co., 1990.
Klaper, Michael, M.D. *Vegan Nutrition: Pure and Simple*. Gentle World, 1987.
McDougall, John, M.D. *The McDougall Program: Twelve Days to Dynamic Health*. NAL-Dutton, 1990.
☆ McDougall, John, M.D. and Mary McDougall. *The McDougall Plan*. New Win Publishing, Inc., 1985.
Ornish, Dean, M.D. *Dr. Dean Ornish's Program for Reversing Heart Disease*. Ballantine Books, 1992.

## Children

Attwood, Charles, M.D. *Dr. Attwood's Low-Fat Prescription for Kids: A Pediatrician's Program of Preventive Nutrition.* Viking-Penguin, 1995.

Klaper, Michael, M.D. *Pregnancy, Children and the Vegan Diet.* Gentle World, 1988.

Yntema, Sharon. *Vegetarian Baby.* McBooks Press, 1991.

_____. *Vegetarian Children.* McBooks Press, 1995.

_____. *Vegetarian Pregnancy.* McBooks Press, 1994.

## Macrobiotics

Ferre, Carl, ed. *Essential Ohsawa.* Avery, 1994.

## Natural Hygiene

Diamond, Harvey with Marilyn Diamond. *Fit for Life II: Living Health.* Warner Books, 1989.

## Raw Foods

Schaeffer, Severen L. *Instinctive Nutrition.* Celestial Arts, 1987.

## Psychology/Sociology

☆ Amato, Paul with Sonia Partridge. *The New Vegetarians.* Plenum Press, 1989.

Burns, David, M.D. *Feeling Good: The New Mood Therapy.* Avon Books, 1980.

Covey, Stephen R. *The Seven Habits of Highly Effective People.* Simon & Schuster, 1989.

Hirschmann, Jane with Carol Munter. *Overcoming Overeating.* Ballantine Books, 1988.

Jeffers, Susan. *Feel The Fear and Do It Anyway.* Ballantine Books, 1987.

McWilliams, Peter. *Do It! Let's Get off Our Buts.* Prelude Press, 1994.

Schwartz, Robert. *Diets Still Don't Work.* Breakthru Publishing, 1990.

Siegel, Michele, with Judith Brisman and Margot Weinshel. *Surviving an Eating Disorder: Strategies for Family and Friends*. Harper & Row, 1988.

## Ethics

Adams, Carol. *The Sexual Politics of Meat*. Continuum Publishing Company, 1991.

Boyd, Billy Ray. *For the Vegetarian in You*. Prima Press, 1996.

Kapleau, Roshi P. *To Cherish All Life: A Buddhist View of Animal Slaughter and Meat Eating*. Zen Center, 1981.

Lappe, Frances Moore. *Diet for a Small Planet*, (20th Anniversary Edition). Ballantine Books, 1991.

Linzey, Andrew. *Christianity and the Rights of Animals*. Crossroad Publishing Co., 1987.

Masri, Al-Hafiz B.A. *Islamic Concern for Animals*. The Athene Trust, 3A Charles St., Peterfield, Hants GU32 3EH, England, 1987. (Send a query with a self-addressed envelope and an International Reply Coupon, available from U.S. post offices.)

☆ Mason, Jim with Peter Singer. *Animal Factories*. Harmony Books, 1990.

Rifkin, Jeremy. *Beyond Beef*. NAL-Dutton, 1992.

☆ Robbins, John. *Diet for a New America*. Stillpoint Publishing, 1987.

Rosen, Steven. *Food for the Spirit: Vegetarianism and the World Religions*. Bala Books, 1987.

Schwartz, Richard. *Judaism and Vegetarianism*. Micah Publications, 1988.

Singer, Peter. *Animal Liberation*. The New York Review of Books, 1990.

Wynne-Tyson, Jon, ed. *The Extended Circle*. Paragon House Publishers, 1989.

## Magazines

*Vegetarian Gourmet*, P.O. Box 10647, Riverton, NJ 08076-0647 (717-278-1984).

*Vegetarian Journal*, The Vegetarian Resource Group, P.O. Box 1463, Baltimore, MD 21203 (410-366-8343).

*Vegetarian Living*, Nexus Media, Greater London House, Hampstead Road, London NW1 7QQ, England (071-388-3171).

☆ *Vegetarian Times* (subscription information: 800-435-9610; outside U.S.: 815-734-5824).

*Veggie Life*, Box 412, Mt. Morris, IL 61054-8163 (800-777-1164).

## Literature

In addition to the above nonfiction works on vegetarianism, I highly recommend the following fiction for an improved understanding of social change, dominionism, and vegetarianism:

### Short Stories
Anthony, Piers. "In The Barn."
Singer, Isaac Bashevis. "The Slaughterer."
Walker, Alice. "Am I Blue?"
_____. "Why Did the Balinese Chicken Cross the Road?"

### Novels
Sinclair, Upton. *The Jungle*.
Stowe, Harriet Beecher. *Uncle Tom's Cabin*.

## *Educational Materials*

### Pamphlets

*Becoming a Vegetarian*. Physicians Committee for Responsible Medicine (202-686-2210).

*Diet and Health: Implications for Reducing Chronic Disease Risk*. National Research Council. National Academy Press, 1989.

*Position Paper on Vegetarianism*. American Dietetic Association (312-877-4815; ask for the Practice department).

*The Surgeon General's Report on Nutrition and Health: Summary and Recommendations*. United States Department of

Health and Human Services. DHHS Public Health Service Publication No. 88-50211, Superintendent of Documents, U.S. Government Printing Office, Washington DC 20402; 1988.

## Cafeteria Food Plan Kits

*The Choice Program from the Farm Animal Reform Movement* (301-5301-1737).
*The Gold Plan from the Physicians Committee for Responsible Medicine* (202-686-2210).
*The Healthy School Lunch Action Guide from the EarthSave Foundation* (800-362-3648).
*Quantity Recipe Packet; Tips for Introducing Vegetarian Food to Institutions* (pamphlet); and *Food Service Quarterly* (newsletter) from the Vegetarian Resource Group (410-366-8343).

## Videos

*The Animals' Film.* The Cinema Guild; 1697 Broadway, Suite 506, NY, NY 10019; (212-246-5522).
*A Diet for All Reasons,* with Michael Klaper, M.D. FARM; Box 30654, Bethesda, MD, 20824.
*Diet for a New America,* with John Robbins. EarthSave Foundation; (408-423-4069).
*Friendly Foods Cooking Techniques,* with Brother Ron Picarski. Eco-Cuisine Inc., 125 Pleasant St., Suite 611, Brookline, MA 02146; (617-738-4363).
*Ten Talents Natural Foods Vegetarian Cuisine: Lifestyle and Nutrition Seminar Series 1-10* (5 tape set), with Dr. Frank Hurd and Rosalie Hurd. Route 1, Box 86A, Chisholm, MN 55719; (218-254-5357).
*Vegan Kitchen,* with Freya Dinshah. American Vegan Society; (609-694-2887).
*The Vegetarian Times Video Series.* Vegetarian Times Magazine; (800-435-9610).

## *Organizations*

### Vegetarian Societies

For local vegetarian societies, look in the phone book or contact one of the national vegetarian groups below for information on groups in your area:

The American Vegan Society
P.O. Box H
Malaga, NJ 08328
609-694-2887

The North American Vegetarian Society
P.O. Box 72,
Dolgeville, NY 13329
518-568-7970

Vegetarian Awareness Network
24-hour message: 800-USA-VEGE

The Vegetarian Resource Group
P.O. Box 1463
Baltimore, MD 21203
410-366-8343

Vegetarian Union of North America
P.O. Box 9710
Washington, DC 20016

### Food Activism

The Abundant Life Seed Foundation
P.O. Box 772
1029 Lawrence St
Port Townsend, WA 98368
206-385-5660

The EarthSave Foundation
706 Frederick St.
Santa Cruz, CA 95062
408-423-4069

The Food First Institute
398 60th St
Oakland, CA 94618
510-654-4400

Food Not Bombs
800-884-1136

The Health Connection
55 West Oak Ridge Drive
Hagerstown, MD 21740-7390
800-548-8700

The Physicians Committee for Responsible Medicine
P.O. Box 6322
Washington DC 20015
202-686-2210

The Pure Food Campaign
202-775-1132

Seeds of Change
P.O. Box 15700
Santa Fe, NM 87506
505-438-8080

The Soyfoods Center
P.O. Box 234
Lafayette, CA 94549-0234
A stamped, self-addressed envelope is requested.

VeganWorld
P.O. Box 2565
Marco Island, FL 33969
941-642-1000

## Animal Rights

Farm Animal Reform Movement
10101 Ashburton Lane
Bethesda, MD 20817
301-530-1737

Compassion in World Farming
20 Lavant St
Petersfield, Hampshire GU32 3EW
England

Feminists for Animal Rights
P.O. Box 694, Cathedral Station
New York, NY 10025
212-866-6422

People for the Ethical Treatment of Animals
P.O. Box 42516
Washington, DC 20015
301-770-7382

United Poultry Concerns, Inc.
P.O. Box 59367
Potomac, MD 20859
301-948-2406

## Alternative Medicine

A good way to find any medical practitioner, of course, is through personal referrals, so you may want to ask trusted friends for the name of a physician who understands vegetarian diets. For further information about "alternative" practitioners in your area, contact the following organizations:

American Association of Naturopathic Physicians
2366 East Lake Avenue, Suite 322
Seattle, WA 98102
206-323-7610

The American Chiropractic Association
1701 Clarendon Blvd.
Arlington, VA 22209
703-276-8800

The American Holistic Medical Association
4101 Lake Boone Trail, Suite 201
Raleigh, NC 27607
919-787-5146

The American Natural Hygiene Society
P.O. Box 30630
Tampa, FL 33630
813-855-6607

The National Center for Homeopathy
801 North Fairfax St., Suite 306
Alexandria, VA 22314
703-548-7790

## Internet

Given the rapidity of change on the Internet, the following list may very well be out of date by the time this book is published! However, a wealth of information about, by, and for vegetarians thrives in the electronic media of e-mail postings, homepages, and newsgroups. If these particular sites are no longer in service, many others will undoubtedly have sprung up to take their place. Key words to use for searches are "vegetarian," "vegan," "animal rights," "diet," "health," "cooking," and "nutrition." Many sites also link to others, and there are several detailed indexes of vegetarian resources on the Net.

## E-mail Resources

Vegan-L: For information on subscribing, send e-mail to "listserv@templevm.bitnet", and include in your message: sub vegan-l and your first and last names.

VegLife: For information on subscribing, send e-mail to "listserv@vtvm1.cc.vt.edu", and include in your message: sub veglife and your first and last names.

Vegetarianism Frequently Asked Questions (FAQ) file: available through Michael Traub at "traub@btcs.bt.co.uk".

AR-TALK: For information on subscribing, send e-mail to "AR-Talk-Request@cygnus.com".

Animal Rights Frequently Asked Questions (FAQ) file: available through Donald Graft at "dgraft@gate.net".

## Newsgroups

For interactive talk about vegetarianism and related issues, contact: "rec.food.veg".

For recipes and cooking information, contact: "rec.food.veg.cooking".

## World Wide Web

Animal Rights Resource Site:
http://www.envirolink.org/arrs/index.html

FAQs about Vegetarianism:
http://www.lib.ox.ac.uk/internet/news/faq/archive/vegetarian

International Vegetarian Union:
http://www.veg.org/veg/Orgs/IVU/

Mega Vegetarian Index:
http://www.macav.chautauqua.com/vegindex.html

Vegan Awakening:
http://www.vegan.org/awakening/

Vegetarian Pages:
http://www.veg.org/veg/

Vegetarian Resource Group:
http://www.envirolink.org/arrs/VRG/home.html

The Vegetarian Society of the United Kingdom:
http://www.veg.org/veg/Orgs/VegSocUK

Veggies Unite—A Searchable Vegetarian Cookbook:
http://www.honors.indiana.edu/~veggie/recipes.cgi

World Guide to Vegetarianism:
http://www.veg.org/veg/Guide/index.html

# Mail-Order Food Sources

Good Eats
Box 756
Richboro, PA 18954-0756
800-490-0044
Over 1500 organic natural foods plus a wide selection of
other ecological products.

Heartland Foods
Route 2, Box 189B
Susquehanna, PA 18847
717-879-8790
Vegetarian foods and organic products.

The Mail Order Catalog
P.O. Box 180
Summertown, TN 38483
800-695-2241
Meat substitutes, nutritional yeast, soymilk powder, and an
    extensive bookshelf.

Natural Way Mills, Inc.
Route 2, Box 37
Middle River, MN 56737
218-222-3677
Organic whole grains and dry-milled grain products.

Phipps Beans
P.O. Box 349
Pescadero, CA 94060
800-279-0889
Dried beans, peas, and lentils.

Timber Crest Farms
4791 Dry Creek Road
Healdsburg, CA 95448
707-433-8251
Dried tomato products, pasta sauces, salsas, dried fruits
    and nuts.

Uncle John's Foods
Box 489
Fairplay, CO 80440
800-530-8733
Dehydrated vegan meals for campers and backpackers.

Vegetarian Gourmet Gift Baskets
Vista International
P.O. Box 546742
Surfside, FL 33154
800-868-9502
Four styles of gift baskets, each containing a wide selection
of vegetarian foods.

Walnut Acres
Walnut Acres Road
Penns Creek, PA 17862
717-837-0601
Organic whole grain cereals, vegetarian soups and chilis,
dried fruits, and other foods.

The Whole Earth Vegetarian Catalog
Lumen Foods
409 Scott St.
Lake Charles, LA, 70601
800-256-2253
Meat substitutes, veggie burgers, soy milk, and other items.

## Vegetarian Pet Food Companies
Harbingers of a New Age
717 East Missoula Ave.
Troy, MT 59935
406-295-4944
Vegepet supplements and recipes.

Natural Life Pet Products
P.O. Box 943
Frontenac, KS 66763
800-367-2391
Vegetarian dog kibble and vegetarian canned dog food.
Call or write to obtain information about your local
distributor.

Nature's Recipe
341 Bonnie Circle
Corona, CA 91720
800-843-4008
Vegetarian dog kibble and vegetarian canned dog food. Call or
write to obtain information about your local distributor.

Wysong
800-748-0188
Vegetarian and vegan kibble designed for cats and dogs
who have allergies. Call to obtain information about
your local distributor.

## Animal-Origin Food Ingredients

*Albumen* (used in baked goods): Egg white.

*Albumin* (used in baked goods, candy, and to clarify wines):
Proteins derived from egg whites, other animal products, and plants.

*Amino acids* (used in vitamins and supplements): The build-
ing blocks of protein, they may be taken from either
plants or animals.

*Animal fats* (used in cooking and baking).

*Bee pollen* (used in supplements): Spores collected from
flowers by bees.

*Bone char* (used to bleach white sugar): A charcoal made
from the ash of animal bones.

*Bone meal* (used in vitamins and supplements, usually as a
calcium source): Finely crushed animal bones.

*Broth* (used in cooking): Liquid in which flesh or plants
have been cooked. Also called "stock."

*Butter* (used in cooking and baking): A substance made by
mixing milk fats and air.

*Carmine* (used as a red food coloring): Dried female cochineal insects.

*Casein* (used in soy dairy products and in baked goods): A protein from cow's milk.

*Cetyl alcohol/palmitate*: A derivative of spermaceti.

*Cheese*: The curds of cow's or goat's milk, which are usually pressed or molded into solid blocks and allowed to ripen.

*Condensed milk* (used in cooking and baking): Evaporated, sweetened milk.

*Cream* (used in cooking and baking as well as in hot drinks): Fats which rise to the top of fresh milk.

*Cystine* (used in baked goods): An amino acid which can be derived from animal tissue.

*Duodenum substances* (used in vitamins): Substances derived from the digestive tracts of animals.

*Eggs* (used in cooking and baking): The ova of birds. They are often separated into the whites and yolks.

*Fatty acids* (used in various foods): Includes linoleic acid and palmitic acid. They can be from animal or plant sources.

*Fish liver oil* (used in vitamins and supplements, including cow's milk fortified with vitamin D): From cod and similar fish.

*Fish oil* (used in shortenings and margarines): From fish or marine mammals.

*Gelatin* (used in vitamins, medicine capsules, puddings, gelatin desserts, marshmallows, and other foods. Also used to clarify wines): A glutinous protein from boiled animal tissues.

*Glycerine* (used in various foods): Either animal or plant fats are mixed with alkali to form soap and its by-product, glycerine.

*Half-and-half* (used in cooking and baking as well as in hot drinks): A mixture of whole milk and cream.

*Honey* (used in baking, in hot drinks, and as a spread): A substance produced by bees from flower nectar.

*Isinglass* (used in foods and to clarify wines): A very pure form of gelatin made from the air bladders of fish.

*Lactic acid* (used in fermented and pickled foods): From fermented carbohydrates such as lactose or plant sugars.

*Lactose* (used in baked goods): A sugar derived from cow's milk.

*Lard* (used in baked goods and other foods): Pig fat.

*Lecithin* (used in candies and other foods): Derived from eggs or soybeans. If the latter, the label will specify "soy lecithin."

*Lipase* (used in vitamins): An enzyme derived from the stomachs and glands of young herbivores such as calves, lambs, and kids.

*Milk* (used in baking and cooking as well as a beverage): A liquid secreted from the mammary glands of a female mammal as food for her baby. Legally, only cow's milk can be called "milk." All other milks and milk-like substances must be preceded by a modifier (eg: goat's milk, soy milk).

*Mono- and di-glycerides* (used in baked goods, candies, margarines, and other foods): Derived from glycerine and therefore from either animal or plant sources.

*Musk oil* (used as a food flavoring): From fur-bearing animals and musk deer.

*Myristic acid* (used as a food flavoring): From animal and plant fats.

*Nucleic acids* (used in vitamins and supplements): From animal and plant cells.

*Oleic acid* (used in various foods): From animal and plant fats, but most often derived from tallow.

*Oyster shell* (used in vitamins and supplements, usually as a calcium source): The crushed shells of oysters.

*Polysorbates* (used in various foods): From fatty acids.

*Propolis* (used in supplements): A tree resin collected by bees.

*Rennet* (used to coagulate dairy products): From the stomach linings of calves.

*Royal jelly* (used in supplements): A secretion of honeybees.

*Shortening* (used in baking): A solid fat of either animal or plant origin.

*Sperm oil or spermaceti* (used in margarines): From marine mammals, plant oils, and synthetics.

*Stearic acid*: A derivative of tallow or other fats.

*Stock* (used in cooking): Liquid in which flesh or plants have been cooked. Also called "broth."

*Sugar* (used in baked goods and other foods): White sugar is bleached through a char of animal bones. Brown sugar is made by adding molasses to white sugar.

*Tallow* (used in margarines): Cow or sheep fat.

*Urea* (used to brown baked goods): From animal urine or synthetics.

*Whey* (used in baked goods): When cow's milk is coagulated, it separates into the solid curds and the liquid whey.

*Whipped cream* (used in baking): Cream that has been mixed with air.

*Wine*: Many wines use eggs, gelatin, or other animal products in the "fining" (clarification) process.

# *Notes*

## Chapter 1. Changing Habits, Changing Lives

1. Vic Sussman, *The Vegetarian Alternative* (Rodale Press, 1978), p. 70.
2. Ibid., pp. 1–2.
3. "Carrot & Stick," *Vegetarian Times*, Oct 1995, p. 20.
4. *Vegetarian Times* magazine poll of 1992.
5. Neal Barnard, M.D., *Food for Life: How the New Four Food Groups Can Save Your Life* (Crown Publishers, 1993), pp. 126-127.
6. John Robbins, *Diet for a New America* (Stillpoint Publishing, 1987), p. 315.
7. Ibid., pp. 309-312.
8. Ibid., pp. 303-305.

9. Neal Barnard, M.D., *The Power of Your Plate* (The Book Publishing Company, 1990), pp. 105-106.
10. Robbins, *Diet for a New America*, pp. 156-163.
11. "News From the Dying Industry," *The Farm Report*, Farm Animal Reform Movement, Summer/Fall 1995, p. 8.
12. Frances Moore Lappe, *Diet for a Small Planet*, 10th Anniversary Edition (Ballantine Books, 1982), p. 66.
13. J. Raloff, "U.N. treaty to aid 'international' fish," *Science News*, December 9, 1995, Vol. 148, No. 24, p. 389.
14. Robbins, *Diet for a New America*, pp. 110-112.
15. Kenneth Russell, revised by Stephen Williams, *The Herdsman's Book* (Farming Press Ltd., 1987).
16. Elspeth Lambert, "Dairy Products: The Milking of Cows," *The Animals' Agenda*, July/Aug 1985.
17. Peter Singer, *Animal Liberation* (Avon Books), pp. 147-154.
18. Robbins, *Diet for a New America*, pp. 135-144.
19. Frances Moore Lappe and Joseph Collins, *Food First: Beyond the Myth of Scarcity* (Institute for Food and Development Policy, 1978), pp. 288-289.
20. Ibid., p. 148.
21. Robbins, *Diet for a New America*, pp. 136-137.
22. Ibid., p. 367.
23. Barnard, *The Power of Your Plate*, pp. 165-175.

## Chapter 3. Fine-tuning

1. Michael Klaper, M.D., *Vegan Nutrition: Pure and Simple* (Gentle World, 1987), p. i.
2. Ibid., p. 4.
3. Jane Hirschmann and Carol Munter, *Overcoming Overeating* (Ballantine Books, 1988), p. 141.
4. Sussman, *The Vegetarian Alternative*, p. 7.
5. Michio Kushi with Stephen Blauer, *The Macrobiotic Way* (Paragon Press, 1993), pp. 61-81.
6. *The Surgeon General's Report on Nutrition and Health: Summary and Recommendations*, U.S. Department of Health and Human Services, Publication No. 88-50211, 1988, p. 9.

7. Barnard, *The Power of Your Plate*, p. 208.
8. McDougall, *The McDougall Plan* (New Century Publishers, 1983), pp. 95-106.
9. Ibid., pp. 100-104.
10. Robbins, *Diet for a New America*, p. 174.
11. Physician's Committee For Responsible Medicine, "Vegetarian Starter Kit," p. 5.
12. Barnard, *The Power of Your Plate*, p. 184.
13. Ibid., p. 184.
14. McDougall, *The McDougall Plan*, pp. 100-106.
15. Ibid., pp. 50, 140.
16. Barnard, *Food for Life*, pp. 43-44.
17. McDougall, *The McDougall Plan*, p. 130.
18. Physicians Committee for Responsible Medicine, "Vegetarian Starter Kit," p. 10.
19. McDougall, *The McDougall Plan*, pp. 39-40.
20. Physicians Committee for Responsible Medicine, "Vegetarian Starter Kit," p. 10.
21. McDougall, *The McDougall Plan*, pp. 130, 136.
22. Ibid., pp. 129-130.

## Chapter 4. Other Considerations

1. Barnard, *Food For Life*, pp. 78.
2. Harbingers of a New Age, *Dogs and Cats Go Vegetarian*.
3. Barnard, *The Power of Your Plate*, p. 162.
4. Hirschmann and Munter, *Overcoming Overeating* (Ballantine Books, 1988), pp. 113-115.
5. Barnard, *The Power of Your Plate*, p. 162.
6. Michelle Siegel, Judith Brisman, and Margot Weinshel, *Surviving an Eating Disorder: Strategies for Family and Friends* (Harper & Row, 1988), pp. 14-15.

# *Index*

For more about vegetarianism, including vegetarian
parenting, visit the McBooks Press website on the
World Wide Web at www.McBooks.com.